Work-Related Upper Limb Disorders

Work-Related Upper Limb Disorders: Recognition and Management

Michael A. Hutson MA MB BChir MAE
Specialist Orthopaedic Physician, The Park Row Clinic, Nottingham, and the Leeds General Infirmary, UK; President of the British Institute of Musculoskeletal Medicine, UK.

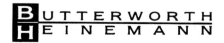

Butterworth-Heinemann
Linacre House, Jordan Hill, Oxford OX2 8DP
225 Wildwood Avenue, Woburn, MA 01801-2041
A division of Reed Educational and Professional Publishing Ltd

 A member of the Reed Elsevier plc group

OXFORD   AUCKLAND   BOSTON
JOHANNESBURG   MELBOURNE   NEW DELHI

First published in 1977
Paperback edition 1999

© Reed Educational and Professional Publishing Ltd 1997

British Library Cataloguing in Publication Data
Hutson, M. A.
    Work-related upper limb disorders: recognition and management
    1. Over-use injuries – Diagnosis   2. Over-use injuries – Treatment
    3. Arm – Wounds and injuries   4. Occupational diseases
    I. Title
    617.4'7'044

Library of Congress Cataloging in Publication Data
Hutson, M. A.
    Work-related upper limb disorders: recognition and management Michael A. Hutson.
    p.   cm.
    Includes bibliographical references and index.
    1. Over-use injuries.   2. Arm – Wounds and injuries.   3. Overexertion injuries.   I. Title.
    [DNLM: 1 Cumulative Trauma Disorders.   2. Musculoskeletal Diseases.
    3. Human Engineering.]
    RD97.6.H88 1997
    617.5'7033–dc21

ISBN 0 7506 4548 2

Typeset by Interactive Sciences Ltd, Gloucester
Printed and bound in Great Britain by
Bookcraft (Bath) Ltd, Midsomer Norton, Somerset

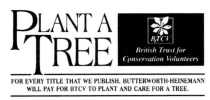

2/24/06

Contents

Preface

There could hardly be a more unbearable – and more irrational – world than one in which the most eminent specialists in each field were allowed to proceed unchecked with the realization of their ideals. F. A. Hayek (1944), *The Road to Serfdom*

There is widespread acceptance that adverse ergonomic factors such as poor postures, bad work practices, frequent repetitive tasks, forceful movements of the hand and arm, and prolonged static loading of the muscles of the neck and shoulders, may have a causal relationship with a number of well-defined musculoskeletal conditions and nerve entrapment syndromes affecting the upper limb. These work-related upper limb disorders are referred to collectively in this book as type 1 WRULDs. Examples of these conditions in which there are positive physical signs and demonstrable organic pathology are de Quervain's tenovaginitis, peritendinitis crepitans, carpal tunnel syndrome, subacromial impingement and lateral epicondylitis.

Type 1 conditions have relatively clear-cut clinical characteristics and established treatment protocols. They are not a homogeneous group, however, and careful assessment is required in individual cases, particularly with respect to the identification of stressors. Causation may be a difficult and contentious issue, but one that affects management, prevention and prognosis as well as litigation. The aetiological factors and histological characteristics are included in the description of these discrete conditions in Chapter 5.

By contrast, a type 2 WRULD is a regional pain syndrome in which there is widespread dissemination of symptoms between the neck and the hand. This relatively intangible condition has sometimes been categorized as a psychosocial phenomenon, somatization, or frank neurosis, capable of developing into epidemic proportions, because of the apparent paucity or absence of meaningful physical signs and recognizable pathology. In this context a frequently expressed view is that the condition is more prevalent in people with vulnerable personalities, but an alternative hypothesis is that it occurs in those with vulnerable neuromuscular constitutions. A discussion on the relative contributions of psychophysiological and neurophysiological disturbances to the development of type 2 WRULD is undertaken in the following chapters.

Regional allodynia and hyperalgesia are characteristic features of type 2 WRULD. Early recognition of the progression from axial or peripheral injury, soft tissue or neural in type, to a state of neural sensitization – frequently precipitated, perpetuated or provoked by adverse psychosocial factors – provides the principal opportunity to abort its development into a refractory chronic pain syndrome.

An important aetiological factor in the progression from early to established type 2 WRULD is iatrogenesis. Errors of diagnosis and management may occur at the first medical contact (usually with the family doctor), when 'teno' is frequently diagnosed (with its connotation of employer culpability) whatever the true nature of the condition. Potentially more serious, however, following secondary referral, is the refutation by the 'specialist' of the possibility of neuromuscular dysfunction on the basis of the lack of hard physical signs (with the implied fabrication of the severity of the condition by the patient).

An established type 2 WRULD is refractory to conventional therapeutic measures that are effective for a traditional disease (or disease–illness) model, and it is not surprising that the sufferer becomes confused and disheartened. Not uncommonly, she (more often than 'he') develops a heightened awareness of her symptoms and increasing anxiety regarding her persistent, and often increasingly intrusive, disability. Secondary psychological manifestations and seemingly 'inappropriate' behavioural responses are common at this stage.

Of major importance to the understanding of the pathogenesis of both type 1 and type 2 WRULDs is the modification of the stringent demands (associated with the 'structuralist' approach) for demonstrable 'organic' pathology by the acknowledgement of the potential roles played by neuroplasticity and neuromuscular dysfunction. The 'functionalist' approach espouses the dynamic, biomechanical and pathophysiological responses of the spine, the nervous system and the soft tissues to repetitive loading. A familiarity with the concept of dysfunction will allow common sense and understanding to prevail over dogma.

Overuse conditions result from overload – that is, they occur when the biological tolerance of the soft tissues to stress is overcome. Our rapidly expanding knowledge of neurogenic mechanisms, particularly the development of the theory of central sensitization (Woolf, 1983) following the seminal work of Melzack and Wall in 1965, should enable the predication of a sound clinical practice around an enlightened musculoskeletal examination. Clinical findings such as allodynia and myofascial trigger points (hyperalgesia) may then be confidently recorded with comprehension of their relevance. Considerable emphasis is placed upon appropriate manual (examination) skills in this text.

One may learn much from a study of the historical perspective – not least because the great neurologists of the late nineteenth century were so observant and analytical, identifying both central and peripheral mechanisms in the pathogenesis of conditions such as scrivener's palsy. By contrast, the more recent (archetypal) Australian view, reflected in the extensive literature on the epidemic of 'RSI' in the 1980s, became very polarized towards the concepts of the disingenuousness of complainants/patients and the maladroitness of the medical profession.

Whilst sympathizing with the contemporaneous Australian hypothesis of the 1980s that control of the epidemic depended upon suppression of the concept of 'injury' or indeed any speculative physical condition that suggested liability, a more appropriate and reflective view in the 1990s should be based on the neurogenic pathogenesis of type 2 WRULD and the validity of the associated psychosocial component. (What medical condition or 'disease' does not have some psychosocial component?) As a corollary, the medical profession should be supportive of industry in the provision of a more attractive and ergonomically sound environment in which a vulnerable workforce may operate with safety.

References

Melzack, R. and Wall, P.D. (1965) Pain mechanisms: a new theory. *Science*, **150**, 971–8.

Woolf, C.J. (1983) Evidence for a central component of post-injury pain hypersensitivity. *Nature*, **306**, 686–8.

1
Historical perspective

Of the neuralgic variety of 'piano-failure': first there is the nerve-tenderness which accompanies almost all of these cases. This may definitely be brought about by over-use of the muscles; it may also occur in connection with a wrench or strain of the arm, or may follow a bruise, and it seems very liable to occur in persons of delicate organization who are in depressed health or who have been exposed to cold.

G. Vivian Poore (1887b).

Plus ça change, plus c'est la même chose

Politicians recognize the value of a sound understanding of the sociopolitical history of their own country, particularly when faced with contemporary problems that appear to be formidable or insoluble. Similarly, a grasp of the historical background to the evolution of contemporary medical views on the upper limb disorders is very instructive (Quintner, 1991). One might conclude that there is little new after reviewing the hypotheses propounded for these conditions over the past one hundred and fifty years.

Scrivener's palsy

Bernadino Ramazzini (1633–1714), the founder of occupational medicine (Figure 1.1), described the problems experienced by scribes (who wrote with a quill) in his treatise *De morbis artificum* in 1713:

furthermore, incessant driving of the pen over paper causes intense fatigue of the hand and the whole arm because of the continuous and almost tonic strain on the muscles and tendons, which in course of time results in failure of power in the right hand ... what tortures these workers most acutely is the intense and incessant application of the mind, for in work such as this the whole brain,

its nerves and fibres, must be constantly on the stretch: hence ensues loss of tonus.

It is clear that Ramazzini was aware of the interaction between mental stress and musculotendinous strain 300 years ago.

In the 1830s there was an outbreak of writer's cramp in male clerks working in the British Civil Service, which was attributed to the introduction of the steel nib in preference to

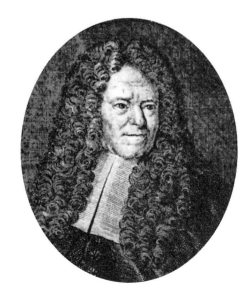

Figure 1.1 Bernadino Ramazzini, the founder of occupational medicine

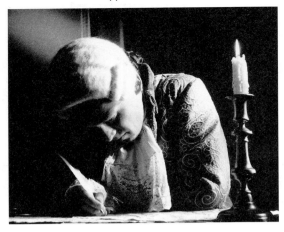

Figure 1.2 Scrivener's palsy (writer's cramp) has been known since Ramazzini described the condition in *De morbis artificum* in 1713. (Courtesy of Jonathan Fisher)

the goose-quill pen. This 'partial paralysis of the muscles of the extremities' was described by Sir Charles Bell in 1833.

Samuel Solly, senior surgeon at St Thomas's Hospital, also wrote on scrivener's palsy, or 'the paralysis of writers' (1864, 1867). He described pain in the thumb and forefinger, fatigue, loss of power, trembling, cramps and radiation of discomfort up the limb; the symptoms tended to be specific to writing (Figure 1.2). He referred to similar conditions described by Virchow – shoemaker's cramp, milking cramp, musician's cramp, compositor's and sempstress' cramp. Solly considered that an injury to a nervous centre, possibly in the spinal cord or the cerebellum, accounted for this condition.

Over the next few decades, scrivener's palsy, subsequently referred to as 'writer's cramp', was described by other workers, notably George Vivian Poore at University College Hospital, London. Poore (1878, 1887a) identified both the spasmodic form of writer's cramp and the neuritic (or neuralgic) form. The former group probably constituted what is now recognized to be a form of (focal) dystonia that is characterized by cramps. The neuritic form, on the other hand, is almost certainly the more diffuse form of work-related upper limb disorder, for which Poore considered there was a peripheral neuromuscular cause. Support for the concept that writer's cramp was primarily a peripheral

neuromuscular condition was forthcoming from Beard (1879) and Paul (1911).

Musician's cramp

Musician's cramp was reported extensively by many authors in the final quarter of the nineteenth century. In a comprehensive historical review undertaken by Fry (1986), it was noted that the condition was described in pianists (Figure 1.3), violinists (in either the fingering hand or the bowing arm, Figure 1.4), cellists, harpists, flautists, percussionists, and zither and guitar players. The predominant symptoms were pain, weakness and loss of fine control; cramp, spasm, reduced cutaneous sensation and proximal radiation of symptoms were also recorded.

Poore (1887b) described pianist's cramp which he preferred to call arm 'failure'. The heterogeneity of the symptoms in the hands and arms of the 21 pianists annotated by Poore suggests that a variety of conditions was being described. One patient clearly suffered from flexor carpi ulnaris tendinitis which was treated by blistering. (Arsenic and the application of strips of capsicum were the alternative remedies that were commonly prescribed.) However, many of the patients had neuralgic symptoms, which were provoked by neural stretch tests that he devised for the median, ulnar and radial nerves. He had also

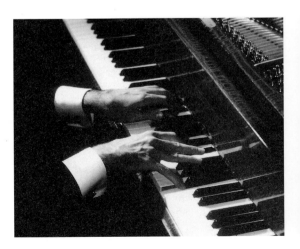

Figure 1.3 Pianists may develop a focal dystonia affecting the fourth and fifth fingers. (Courtesy of Clive Barda)

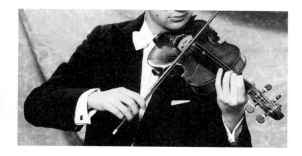

Figure 1.4 Focal dystonia is often lateralized to the fingering (left hand) in string players, but other upper limb disorders may affect the bowing arm too. (Courtesy of Peter Mares)

noted pain on other tests (such as pain over the distal radius on forcible flexion of the thumb) that bear a remarkable resemblance to eponymous tests that are used currently.

Haward (1887) stated that 'in the majority of cases of failure of the muscles of piano-playing, which occur without obvious disease or injury, overuse of the muscles will be found to be the essential cause', a view with which Fry concurred a century later.

Occupational neurosis

At more or less the same time, William Gowers (1845–1915) (Figure 1.5), neurologist at University College Hospital, also wrote on writer's cramp and similar conditions (Gowers, 1892). He used the term 'occupational neurosis' as 'a convenient designation for a group of maladies in which certain symptoms are excited by the attempt to perform some often-repeated muscular action, commonly one that is involved in the occupation of the sufferer'. He was aware of both the motor (spasmodic) and sensory (neuralgic) variety of occupational neurosis and he was aware too that they were particularly common in those of 'nervous' temperament. Gowers considered that anything which lowered the tone of the nervous system acted as a predisposing cause, identifying anxiety as a common associate. Nevertheless, he was prepared to accept that a peripheral neuromuscular disturbance could be a secondary manifestation of what he considered to be a *primary central nervous system*

'derangement'. The frequent bilateral spread of symptoms from the dominant limb appeared to favour a central mechanism.

Oppenheim (1901) in Germany also believed that writer's cramp and other occupational neuroses resulted from a disturbance of the higher centres of the central nervous system, functional rather than organic, in patients with a 'neuropathic' predisposition.

In summary, the dominant *fin de siècle* view appeared to be that occupational neuroses were a form of 'nervous disease – the consequence of the innate vulnerability of the human nervous system to the stresses and strains of civilization' (Drinka, 1984). In retrospect, however, the use of the term 'occupational neurosis' by Gowers to describe a non-organic disturbance of the higher centres of the central nervous system which was

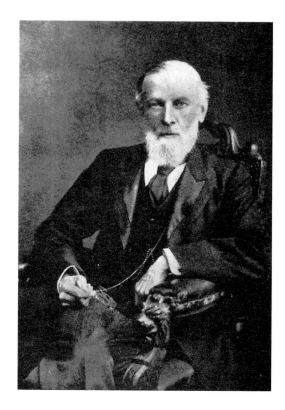

Figure 1.5 Sir William Gowers (1892) used the term 'occupational neurosis' to describe writer's cramp and similar conditions

probably associated with peripheral neural manifestations created some later (twentieth century) confusion. 'Neurosis' subsequently became synonymous with psychoneurosis (which was defined by Freud some time later). However, a generally accepted interpretation of occupational neurosis is that the term as originally used was intended to describe what we now recognize as a neurogenic rather than a psychogenic disturbance.

Telegraphist's cramp

An editorial in *The Lancet* in 1875 headed 'A telegraphic malady' referred to telegraphist's cramp, and added it to the list of diseases that were known as 'professional impotences'. Further reference was made to writer's cramp, hammer palsy (of smiths), sempstress' palsy ('in which the power of plying the needle is lost'), milker's cramp (amongst the cowherds of the Tyrol), and bricklayer's cramp. Interestingly, on comparing the described afflictions in different occupations, the author opined that *'constant repetition does not seem to induce the state of chronic fatigue so quickly as sustained contraction*, because in constantly repeated muscular contraction the muscle enjoys an interval of relaxation, and it is in this interval that its nutrition is maintained'.

Following an outbreak of cramp in telegraphists in the British Isles in the early part of the twentieth century, a Departmental Committee of the Great Britain and Ireland Post Office was set up to study the causes. In its report on telegraphist's cramp in 1911, the conclusion was that the 'nervous breakdown' known as telegraphist's cramp was due to a combination of two factors: one, a nervous 'instability' on the part of the operator, and the other, repeated fatigue during the complicated movements required for sending messages. At that time, it was clear that the association between peripheral pathology and a nervous disposition was recognized.

'Teno'

Velpeau (1825) used the term 'tenosynovitis' in his treatise *Anatomie Chirurgicale*. The term 'washerwoman's sprain' was described in *Gray's Anatomy* of 1893. It is probable that the condition now recognized as peritendinitis crepitans was being described. 'Tendovaginitis crepitans' in the forearm was described in some detail in 1918 by Troell, who compared it to lesions affecting the tendons of the anterior and posterior compartments of the lower leg. Thompson used the term *'peritendinitis crepitans'* in 1951 for the condition now also referred to as intersection syndrome of the forearm.

The Swiss surgeon de Quervain described the condition of 'fibrose, stenosierende tendovaginitis' in 1895. He subsequently described the successful management of a small series of cases by surgery. The same condition referred to as tenosynovitis crépitante had been described by Tillaux in the *Traité d'Anatomie Topographique* in 1892.

Finkelstein (1930) reported on 24 cases, the majority of which, in his opinion, were caused by chronic trauma. He described the eponymous test in which the patient's pain was reproduced when the thumb was placed across the palm, the fist was firmly closed by flexion of the fingers, and the wrist ulnar deviated.

Hyperalgesia

The concept of 'fibrositis' was defined in the early part of the twentieth century by Gowers (1904), who described a painful inflammatory disorder of muscle spindles. Ubiquitously the fibrositic inflammation was considered to be capable of spreading to other soft tissues, to the extent that tenderness over joints, muscles, bursae and nerves was explained on the basis of fibrositic nodules, panniculitis and polyneuritis. Gowers stressed the sensitivity of the musculotendinous structures which were symptomatic when firmly palpated. He described syndromes affecting the neck, pectoral girdle and arm as well as 'lumbago'.

Despite criticism by Cyriax (1941), who considered that referred pain and tenderness were manifestations of extrasegmental reference from dural irritation, the concept of myofascial pain in the shoulder and arm has endured and was expanded upon by Travell as long ago as 1942. Referred pain from muscle had already been described by Kellgren (1938), but Travell developed the concept of myofascial pain by defining the 'myofascial pain syndrome', in which hypertonic trigger points were the essential feature. *The Trigger Point Manual* (Travell and Simons, 1983) has achieved almost biblical respect among sections of the physiotherapy profession over the past decade.

A contrasting opinion, which is based on the concept of a neuropathic pathogenesis of some types of upper limb pain, has been proposed by Quintner and Cohen (1994), who consider that the phenomenon of trigger points is better understood as secondary hyperalgesia of peripheral nerve origin.

Peripheral nerve entrapment

Pfeffer *et al.* (1988) reported that James Putnam, a Boston (USA) neurologist, was the first to describe non-traumatic pain, paraesthesiae and numbness in the median nerve distribution of the hand in 1880, 'possibly of vasomotor origin'. Thirty-seven patients, mainly women with an average age of approximately 35 years, suffered from 'numbness, recurring periodically, coming on especially at night . . . very often excessively intense, so as to amount to real pain in itself . . . in some cases simply letting the arm hang out of the bed or shaking it about for some moments would drive the numbness away'.

In 1909 James Ramsey Hunt of Columbia University attributed thenar atrophy to compression of the motor branch of the median nerve beneath the transverse carpal ligament which resulted from 'occupational over-use'. Subsequently (Hunt, 1911), he explained that the associated sensory symptoms, numbness and paraesthesiae of the fingers were in the nature of an 'acroparaesthesia'. Oppenheim (1901) identified laundry workers, joiners, locksmiths and carpet beaters amongst those occupations in which median nerve pareses were common; he appeared not to appreciate that the carpal tunnel might be the site of entrapment.

At more or less the same time, Marie and Foix (1913) reported on bilateral thenar atrophy that resulted from compression of the median nerve beneath the transverse carpal ligament. Although, according to Pfeffer, they suggested that 'transection of the ligament

could stop the development of these phenomena', their prescience was ignored for several decades.

Eventually, the influence of Learmonth (1933) and Brain *et al.* (1947) prompted the development of the concept of non-traumatic surgically treatable median nerve compression in the carpal tunnel. Finally, Phalen *et al.* (1950) championed the association between median nerve compression and chronic tenosynovitis.

During the 1940s and 1950s the art of nerve conduction as a diagnostic tool for peripheral nerve lesions was developed. A prolonged distal latency following stimulation of the median nerve at the wrist in carpal tunnel syndrome was described by Simpson (1956). Since then the use of electrodiagnosis, particularly the development of sensory action potential recording, has expanded and has become a routine investigative procedure.

Epidemiological studies in the 1970s

Although there have been few epidemiological studies of work-related upper limb disorders that have been carefully constructed by reference to control groups of subjects, the plethora of articles in the medical journals in the 1970s and 1980s were valuable to the extent that they gave an indication of the prevalence of conditions affecting the neck and the upper limb.

In Japan there had been sufficient concern regarding work-related problems for the Japanese Ministry of Labour to introduce work guidelines in 1964. These included frequent rest periods and maximal work intensities. The Japanese Association of Industrial Health created the Committee on Occupational Cervicobrachial Syndrome in 1971. The Committee reported on the condition that was termed 'occupational cervicobrachial disorder' (OCD) in 1973, describing it as 'a disease closely related to the complex of chronic physical fatigue in the neck, shoulders, back, arms and hands, and chronic mental fatigue though this description is to some degree variable, depending on the characteristics of each task'. The number of workers in private industries who were compensated for these disorders increased from 90 to 546 between 1970 and 1975 (Maeda, 1977).

Ohara *et al.* (1976) reported on the incidence of shoulder, arm, wrist and hand symptoms in cash register operators, describing differences with office machine operators and other office workers in Japan. Nagira *et al.* (1981) identified an increased prevalence of disorders affecting the upper limb in certain occupations that demand rapid, repetitive movements. *Hunter's Diseases of Occupations* (Hazelman, 1974) states that an *epidemic* of occupational cervicobrachial disorders was reported in Japan between 1958 and 1992. Workers affected included punch card operators, typists, telephone operators, keyboard operators and process workers.

The term OCD (occupational cervicobrachial disorder) was used in Germany and Scandinavia too. An increase in disorders of the upper limb giving rise to localized discomfort, stiffness and fatigue in the neck and arms was reported in accounting machine operators in Switzerland (Hunting *et al.*, 1980; Maeda *et al.*, 1980). Tenosynovitis and other injuries of the upper extremities in occupations that demand repetitive movements were also described in Finland (Lupoajarvi *et al.*, 1979).

In the UK, tenosynovitis has been a DHSS prescribed disease known as PD 34 (subsequently retitled PD A8), 'at least since 1947' (Semple, 1986). In 1977 the Health and Safety Executive published Guidance Note MS10 describing tenosynovitis as the second commonest prescribed (industrial) disease in the UK, occurring among factory workers and others doing repetitive tasks. According to Semple, its reported prevalence probably arises from the diagnosis (of uncertain accuracy) made by general practitioners on sickness certificates. The Health and Safety Executive statistics for 1981 recorded 2957 claims for industrial injury benefit caused by RSI or similar disorders (HSE, 1982). (For a definition of RSI, see next section.)

The 1980s: the Australian outbreak of RSI

An alarming increase in incidence of RSI amongst data processing operators, accounting machinists and typists employed by the Australian Board of Statistics was recorded in 1981/2 compared with 1975/6. Interestingly, there was considerable geographical variation throughout Australia. There was a significant increase in claims from injury and pain (including RSI) in data processing operators employed in Australian taxation offices between 1980 and 1984 in comparison with the period between 1974 and 1979.

In New South Wales the number of successful occupational claims for RSI (excluding those from the Australian public service) increased from 762 in 1978/9 to 2263 in 1981/2 (McDermott, 1986). There was a 275% increase in the incidence of RSI in the period June 1983 to June 1984 in the Commonwealth Banking Corporation (Task Force, 1985). According to the Task Force statistics, the estimated cost of lost work from July 1984 to June 1985 in the Australian Commonwealth Public Service (excluding state public servants and private enterprise employees) was 24.13 million Australian dollars.

On reviewing the epidemiological aspects of RSI in Telecom Australia in 1987, Hocking stated that nearly 4000 reports of RSI (76% of which involved loss of time from work) were made over the 5 years 1981 to 1985. The incidence peaked in the December 1984 and March 1985 quarters (Figure 1.6). The average time lost from work was 74 days. Reviews of epidemiological studies and aetiological factors were conducted by McDermott (1986) and Ireland (1988). Chatterjee (1987) reflected upon the nature of 'RSI', stating that this was 'an umbrella term . . . consisting of the soft tissue disorders involving the tendons, nerves and the periarticular structures in the upper extremity and neck'. Clearly, a nosological classification was long overdue at that time.

The term RSI, denoting repetitive strain injury or repetition strain injury, was coined by Stone in 1983, although Ferguson (1971) had previously described the same condition in Australian telegraphists and labelled it 'occupational myalgia'. Several theories were put forward to explain the apparent epidemic of upper limb pain in Australian workers in the 1980s. Retrospectively, some of these hypotheses appear somewhat bizarre, yet the strains of imposing order in circumstances that were contemporaneously described as an

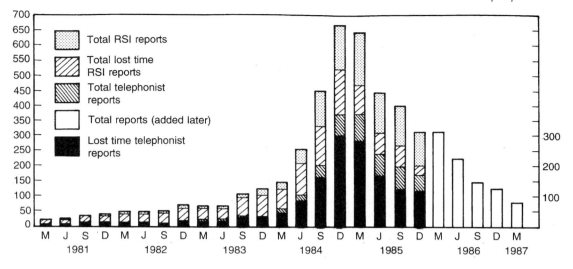

Figure 1.6 Hocking reported on cases of 'RSI' in Telecom Australia between 1981 and 1987. The incidence peaked in the December 1984 and March 1985 quarters. (Based on data from Hocking, 1987)

'epidemic' could explain some of the reasoning behind them.

1 Iatrogenesis

Awerbuch (1986) considered that the readiness of medical practitioners to diagnosis RSI was a principal cause of the epidemic. He stated that 'abnormal diagnosis behaviour leads to abnormal illness behaviour in the patient and is invariably compounded by abnormal treatment behaviour'. In a letter to the *Medical Journal of Australia* in 1985 he was highly critical of the Australian medical profession, lambasting it for contributing to the perpetuation of the epidemic of 'Kangaroo paw' (Figure 1.7), the diagnosis of which rested upon 'only one clinical criterion: namely, the complete absence of objective clinical signs of abnormality'.

The theme of abnormal diagnosis behaviour was taken up by other medical specialists, who may have been disadvantaged to the extent that they did not have a background of expertise in musculoskeletal medicine.

2 Social iatrogenesis

Cleland (1987) considered that cases of RSI were 'diseases caused by a broad range of societal inputs – in the form of statements and publications from official and lay sources

designed to increase awareness and knowledge of potential problems'. However well meant were official statements and information for the lay public, Cleland and others believed that this material was propaganda in the pursuit of litigation.

3 Psychogenic

Somatization, conversion disorder, hysterical neurosis and unrecognized depression or psychosis are quoted by Lucire (1986) as the types

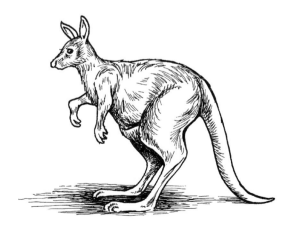

Figure 1.7 Awerbuch lambasted the Australian medical profession for contributing to the perpetuation of the epidemic of 'Kangaroo paw'

of psychogenic illness that may masquerade as work-related upper limb disorder. However, she considered that most claimants had a compensation neurosis and that the epidemic was effectively an **epidemic of hysteria**. She stated that 'the management of such epidemics [of hysteria] is a public health problem which demands community and institutional support as well as co-operation by the media'. She based her judgement as much on the fact that no physical cause had been found for the conditions as on the presence of intrinsic features of neurosis. She stated that 'the search for local pathology in occupational neurosis has yielded no results in 150 years; thus, treatable organic causes now appear improbable'.

Lucire was influential, despite warnings by other authorities regarding the risks of making such a diagnosis. Merskey (1988) cautioned against the diagnosis of psychiatric illness merely in the absence of signs of physical disease. Patrick Wall (1986) stated that 'we need to proceed step by step from the periphery through the afferent nerves and through neuronal circuits of the central nervous system before assuming a psychiatric diagnosis for those patients whose peripheral tissues seem to provide an inadequate basis for their complaint'.

The epistemological flaw in the concept of a primary psychogenic basis for RSI is the failure to distinguish between primary psychological processes (conversion disorder; obsessive, depressive or hysterical neurosis; somatization etc.) and secondary affective features such as reactive depression, frustration, isolation and anger at what are perceived as inadequate medical responses.

4   The illness of work incapacity

Nortin Hadler (1985, 1986) has been a leading figure in the medical campaign against identifying RSI as a credible concept. He invented the phrase 'the facile acronym of RSI' which has been quoted frequently by other authors. He stated that

the medical opinions which supported RSI did not merely lack objective backing, they contradicted established medical knowledge . . . the absence of discrete inflammatory signs renders diagnoses such as de Quervain's disease or other inflammatory tenosynovitis heuristic assertions . . . the pathophysiology of the upper extremity use associated

discomfort is indeterminate . . . the symptom complex defies current nosology.

He considered that the epidemic was due principally to the conversion of indisposition (in the form of aches and pains to which the whole of humanity is subject) to work incapacity, poor coping skills and litigation. The medical and legal professions were largely to blame.

5   Fibrositis syndrome

Littlejohn (1986) identified the condition in which the predominant features were diffuse musculoskeletal aching, dysaesthesiae and tender points in the neck, shoulder and arm as a regional pain syndrome. He equated this to a localized fibrositis syndrome, noting as common denominators (when compared with the generalized fibrositis or fibromyalgia syndrome) the female predisposition, sleep disturbances and 'neuropsychiatric' phenomena. Whilst recognizing the multifactorial nature of the cause of the Australian 'epidemic localized fibrositis syndrome', emphasis was placed on psychosocial, medicolegal and medical management factors.

6   An epidemic of complaints: the archetypal 1980s Australian view

David Ferguson, Emeritus Professor, University of Sydney, in his article 'RSI: putting the epidemic to rest' (1987), stated that 'with hindsight the gigantic and costly Australian epidemic caused by RSI can be seen as a complex psychosocial phenomenon with elements of mass hysteria, that were superimposed on a basis of widespread discomfort, fatigue and morbidity'.

During this period, Peter Brooks (1989) was outspoken. He stated that 'it is clear that the majority of patients with chronic pain *have only that* – they do not have any signs of inflammation or injury' (my italics). It is to be hoped that this attitude was not meant to be as dismissive, arrogant and patronizing as it now sounds in isolation.

Ireland (1988) too was extremely critical of the concept of RSI. His views as a hand surgeon echoed those of his British counterparts. Ireland stated that there are no primary objective physical findings in the upper limb other than tenderness which is frequently of equal severity at any randomly selected point on the limb (*sic*) . . . these conditions are non-physical occupation neuroses . . . the scientific basis of modern medicine demands that diseases are caused by a pathological process which, if not identifiable, has a rational hypothesis, thus enabling formulation and instigation of appropriate management. . . . RSI now bears the hallmark of a sociopolitical phenomenon, rather than a medical condition, which on historical precedent will decline when this basis of RSI is generally accepted.

Current concepts: the 1990s

1 The archetypal (British) hand surgeon's view of RSI

Barton *et al.* (1992) made a definitive statement on behalf of the British Orthopaedic Association in their article 'Occupational causes of disorders in the upper limb' in the *British Medical Journal*. This was a précis of a report prepared on behalf of the BOA for submission to the Industrial Injuries Advisory Council in 1990. Of RSI, Barton *et al.* made the following statements.

- It has not been defined clinically by recognizable signs and symptoms.
- It has no identifiable pathological process.
- The characteristic pain in the arm does not conform to any identifiable anatomical pattern.
- Ireland attributed much of the malady to boredom in people with badly paid, monotonous jobs.
- Hadler held the view that dystrophic or inflammatory changes have seldom if ever been described.

Barton (1989) alleged that, when considering diseases caused by typing and similar conditions of the upper limb,

abnormal physical signs are transient or absent, and there are no objective tests, so accurate diagnosis is often impossible . . . aches and pains are often part of the thousand natural shocks that flesh is heir to . . . apart from peritendinitis crepitans these are diseases without a pathology.

It is clear that the contemporary hand surgeon's view is that the absence of an organic (histopathological) background indicates that there is no physical basis for these conditions. Equally clear is the failure of the orthodox biomedical model of disease to explain the problems of keyboard users and others. Clinicians are trained to consider symptoms and to identify pathology, and often find that concepts such as chronic pain syndromes lie outside their comfort zones.

2 'Repetitive strain injury': semantics or the vernacular?

As a result of the criticisms previously described, particularly the criticism that an epidemic of work-related upper limb pain litigation may be provoked by the use of terminology that could be considered to be inflammatory in this context, the term 'repetitive strain injury' came into disrepute. 'RSI' has been criticized on the basis that the strain is often not a result of 'repetitive' activity but of static muscle loading; that, strictly speaking, there is no identifiable tissue 'strain'; and that the term 'injury' implies culpability on the part of the employer.

It is perfectly true that static muscle loading and constrained postures are probably as important in the development of the diffuse form of WRULD as repetitious activities. However, the criticisms with respect to strain and injury have been levelled principally by clinicians who have not taken account of neural pathogenesis. Accordingly, Pheasant (1994) stated that the argument concerning the meaning of the word 'injury' was 'at best a trivial exercise in semantics and at worst a piece of deliberate obfuscation'. Indeed, the whole argument regarding the use of the term RSI may be criticized as a redundant exercise as it is clear that, in Britain at least, the term continues in common usage.

3 Iatrogenesis: an alternative view

Clinicians have been criticized for making a presumptive diagnosis of RSI 'when no physical condition exists' and thereby fanning the flames of dissatisfaction and litigation in the minds of patients. An alternative view is that far more dissatisfaction and frustration arise as a result of the denial by an intransigent yet influential body of medical opinion of the existence of the condition simply on the basis of a lack of histopathological confirmation.

Iatrogenic disease, manifesting as psychological stress, abnormal illness behaviour and chronic disability, may result from epistemological errors and lack of medical expertise. The outcome of individual patients' problems is often very sensitively balanced at the time of their initial consultation with those medical specialists who undertake (willingly or unwillingly) the responsibility for their management following referral by their general practitioners. (See also 'Epistemological flaws', Chapter 2.)

4 'Occupational overuse syndrome': the archetypal New Zealand view

The term 'occupational overuse syndrome' (OOS) is now used in New Zealand in the same way that WRULD is used in this text. The NZ Occupational Safety and Health Service of the Department of Labour has promoted the concept of prolonged excessive muscle tension as the basis for the overuse variant of OOS. The favoured hypothesis for the **early** stages of the painful symptoms of the diffuse syndrome is a rise in local intramuscular pressure (as a result of maintained muscle tension) and consequent ischaemia. Muscle spasm leads to secondary muscle tension, thence to a self-sustaining cycle of pain. Accordingly, the advocated method of prevention is **relaxation**: work organization, educational and training aspects are promoted in addition to ergonomic considerations and relaxation techniques (Wigley *et al.*, 1992). If the condition progresses, a chronic pain syndrome (along the lines proposed by Cohen *et al.*, 1992) may be superimposed with secondary sympathetic and dystrophic effects.

5 Neuroplasticity

Current concepts regarding neural plasticity and, specifically, the relationship between soft tissue or neural injury and neuropathia are not dissimilar to the concepts of occupational neurosis expressed over one hundred years ago. However, Wall (1991) and Woolf (1991) have elucidated the principal neurophysiological characteristics of physiological pain and pathological pain.

Cohen *et al.* (1992) defined the proposed pathogenesis of what they called 'refractory cervicobrachial pain' (RCBP) syndrome. They realized that 'the Australian RSI phenomenon was an epidemic exaggeration of an endemic complaint'. They proposed that RCBP is 'a reflex neuropathic state consequent upon continuing afferent barrage from nociceptors and mechanoreceptors in anatomically relevant sites. These sites may be in the spinal zygapophyseal joints or related structures, or muscles, tendons, and joint capsules in the upper limb and/or the dorsal root, the dorsal root ganglion or peripheral nerves'. On the question of the (commonly) observed behavioural characteristics associated with regional pain, Cohen considered that abnormal illness behaviour is not a psychiatric illness *per se* but 'a spectrum of maladaptive responses to one's health state, in which sociocultural factors play an important role'.

Summarizing the current view concerning chronic pain and its outward manifestations, pain behaviour is a frequently observed but not inevitable consequence of neuropathic pain. Frankly abnormal illness behaviour develops in some patients with regional pain syndromes such as the diffuse form of WRULD, predominantly as a result of iatrogenic and sociocultural factors. In other words, patients who develop a chronic pain syndrome not only suffer from neurosensitization but are at considerable risk of developing a maladaptive response to environmental stresses too.

References

Anon. (1875) A telegraphic malady (Editorial). *Lancet*, 24 April.

Awerbuch, M. (1985) RSI, or 'Kangaroo paw' (Letter). *Med. J. Aust.*, **142**, 237–8.

Awerbuch, M. (1986) RSI. *Med. J. Aust.*, **145**, 362–3.

Barton, N. (1989). Repetitive strain disorder: often misdiagnosed and often not work related (Editorial). *Br. Med. J.*, **299**, 405–6.

Barton, N.J., Hooper, G., Noble, J. and Steele, W.N. (1992) Occupational causes of disorders in the upper limb. *Br. Med. J.*, **304**, 309–11.

Beard, G.M. (1879) Conclusions from the study of 125 cases of writer's cramp and allied affections. *The Medical Record*, **15**, 244–7.

Bell, C. (1833) Partial paralysis of the muscles of the extremities. In: *The Nervous System of the Human Body*. Duff Green, Washington, DC.

Brain, W.R., Wright, A.D. and Wilkinson, M.C. (1947) Spontaneous compression of both median nerves in the carpal tunnel. Six cases treated surgically. *Lancet*, **i**, 277–82.

Brooks, P. (1989) RSI – regional pain syndrome: the importance of nomenclature. *Br. J. Rheumatol.*, **28**, 180–2.

Chatterjee, D.S. (1987) Repetition strain injury – a recent review. *J. Soc. Occup. Med.*, **37**, 100–5.

Cleland, L.G. (1987) RSI: a model of social iatrogenesis. *Med. J. Aust.*, **147**, 236–9.

Cohen, M.L., Arroyo, J.F., Champion, G.D. and Browne, C.D. (1992) In search of the pathogenesis of refractory cervicobrachial pain syndrome. *Med. J. Aust.*, **156**, 432–6.

Cyriax, J. (1941) *Massage, Manipulation and Local Anaesthesia*. Hamilton, London.

Departmental Committee of Great Britain and Ireland Post Office (1911) Report on telegraphist's cramp. HMSO, London.

Drinka, G.F. (1984) *The Birth of Neurosis: Myth, Malady and the Victorians*. New York, Simon and Schuster.

Ferguson, D. (1971). An Australian study of telegraphist's cramp. *Br. J. Ind. Med.*, **28**, 280–5.

Ferguson, D. (1987) RSI: putting the epidemic to rest. *Med. J. Aust.*, **147**, 213–14.

Finkelstein, H. (1930) Stenosing tendovaginitis at the radial styloid process. *J. Bone Jt Surg.*, **12**, 509–40.

Fry, H.J.H. (1986) Overuse syndrome in musicians – 100 years ago. *Med. J. Aust.*, **145**, 620–5.

Gowers, W.R. (1892) *A Manual of Diseases of the Nervous System*, 2nd edn. J&A Churchill, London, pp. 710–30; also pp. 97–101.

Gowers, W.R. (1904) Lumbago: its lessons and analogues. *Br. Med. J.*, **1**, 117–21.

Hadler, N. (1985) Illness in the workplace: the challenge of musculoskeletal symptoms. *J. Hand Surg.*, **10A**, 451–6.

Hadler, N. (1986) Industrial rheumatology: the Australian and New Zealand experiences with arm pain and backache in the workplace. *Med. J. Aust.*, **144**, 191–5.

Haward, W. (1887) Note on pianist's cramp. *Br. Med. J.*, **1**, 672.

Hazelman, B.L. (1974) Repeated movements and repeated trauma. In: *Hunter's Diseases of Occupations*, 8th edn (eds P.A.B. Raffle *et al.*), London, Arnold, pp. 515–29.

Hocking, B. (1987) Epidemiological aspects of repetition strain injury in Telecom Australia. *Med. J. Aust.*, **147**, 218–22.

HSE (1982) *Health and Safety Statistics, 1981*. Health and Safety Executive, London.

Hunt, J.R. (1909) Occupation neuritis of the thenar branch of the median nerve: a well defined type of atrophy of the hand. *Trans. Am. Neurol. Assoc.*, **35**, 184.

Hunt, J.R. (1911) The thenar and hypothenar types of neural atrophy of the hand. *Am. J. Med. Sci.*, **141**(2), 224.

Hunting, W., Grandjean, E. and Maeda, K. (1980) Constrained postures in accounting machine operators. *Appl. Ergon.*, **11**, 145–9.

Ireland, D.C.R. (1988). Psychological and physical aspects of occupational arm pain. *J. Hand Surg.*, **13B**, 5–10.

Kellgren, J.H. (1938) Observations on referred pain arising from muscle. *Clin. Sci.*, **3**, 175–90.

Learmonth, J.R. (1933) The principle of decompression in the treatment of certain diseases of peripheral nerves. *Surg. Clin. North Am.*, **13**, 905–13.

Littlejohn, G.O. (1986) Repetitive strain syndrome: an Australian experience. *J. Rheumatol.*, **13**(6), 1004–6.

Lucire, Y. (1986) Neurosis in the workplace. *Med. J. Aust.*, **145**, 323–7.

Lupoajarvi, T., Kuorinka, I., Virolainen, M. and Holmberg, M. (1979) Prevalence of tenosynovitis and other injuries of the upper extremities in repetitive work. *Scand. J. Environ. Health*, **5**(3), 48–55.

Maeda, K. (1977) Occupational cervicobrachial disorder and its causative factors. *J. Human Ergol. (Tokyo)*, **6**, 193–202.

Maeda, K., Hunting, W. and Grandjean, E. (1980) Localised fatigue in accounting-machine operators. *J. Occup. Med.*, **22**(12), 810–16.

Marie, P. and Foix, C. (1913) Atrophie isolée de l'éminence thenar d'origine neuritique: rôle du ligament annulaire antérieur du carpe dans la pathogenie de la lesion. *Revue Neurology (Paris)*, **26**, 647–9.

McDermott, F.T. (1986) Repetition strain injury: a review of current understanding. *Med. J. Aust.*, **144**, 196–200.

Merskey, H. (1988) Regional pain is rarely hysterical. *Arch. Neurol.*, **45**, 915–18.

Nagira, T., Suzuki, J., Oi, Y. *et al.* (1981) Cervicobrachial and low back disorders among school lunch workers and nursery school teachers in comparison with cash register operators. *J. Human Ergol. (Tokyo)*, **10**, 117–24.

Ohara, H., Aroyama, H. and Itani, T. (1976) Health hazard among cash register operators and the effects of improved working conditions. *J. Human Ergol. (Tokyo)*, **5**, 31–40.

Oppenheim, H. (1901) *Diseases of the Nervous System*, 1st American edn. J.B. Lippincott Co., London, pp. 807–12.

Paul, W.E. (1911) The aetiology of the occupation neuroses and neuritidies. *J. Nerv. Ment. Dis.*, **38**, 449–66.

Pfeffer, G.B., Gelberman, R.H., Boyes, J.H. and Rydevik, B. (1988) The history of carpal tunnel syndrome. *J. Bone Jt Surg.*, **13B**(1), 28–34.

Phalen, G.S., Garner, W.J., Lalonde, A.A. (1950) Neuropathy of the median nerve due to compression beneath the transverse carpal ligament. *J. Bone Jt Surg.*, **32A**(1), 109–12.

Pheasant, S. (1994) Repetitive strain injury – towards a clarification of the points at issue. *J. Personal Injury Litigation*, September, pp. 223–30.

Poore, G.V. (1878) An analysis of 75 cases of 'writer's cramp' and impaired writing power. *Medico-Chir. Trans.*, **61**, 111–45.

Poore, G.V. (1887a) An analysis of ninety-three cases of writer's cramp and impaired writing power, making, with 75 cases previously reported, a total of 168 cases. Abstract: Proceedings of the Royal Medical and Chirurgical Society. *Lancet*, **ii**, 935–6.

Poore, G.V. (1887b) Clinical lecture on certain conditions of the hand and arm which interfere with performance of professional acts, especially piano playing. *Br. Med. J.*, **1**, 441–4.

de Quervain, F. (1895) Ueber eine form von chronischer tendovaginitis. (Correspondenz – Blatt F.) *Schweizer Arzte*, **25**, 389–94.

Quintner, J. (1991) The RSI syndrome in historical perspective. *Int. Disabil. Stud.*, **13**, 99–104.

Quintner, J.L. and Cohen, M.L. (1994) Referred pain of peripheral nerve origin: an alternative to the 'myofascial pain' construct. *Clin. J. Pain*, **10**, 243–51.

Ramazzini, B. (1713). *De morbis artificum diatriba*. Padua. (Trans. W.C. Wright (1940) in *Diseases of Workers*, Hafner Publishing Co. Inc., New York.)

Semple, C. (1986) Tenosynovitis. *J. Hand Surg.*, **11B**(2), 115–16.

Simpson, J.A. (1956) Electrical signs in the diagnosis of carpal tunnel and related syndromes. *J. Neurol. Neurosurg. Psychiat.*, **19**, 275–80.

Solly, S. (1864) Scrivener's palsy, or the paralysis of writers. *Lancet*, **2**, 709–11.

Solly, S. (1867). On Scrivener's palsy. *Lancet*, **i**, 561–2.

Stone, W.E. (1983) Repetitive strain injuries. *Med. J. Aust.*, **2**, 616–18.

Task Force (1985) *Repetition Strain Injury in the Australian Public Service*. AGPS, Canberra.

Thompson, A.R., Plewes, L.W. and Shaw, E.G. (1951) Peritendinitis crepitans and simple tenosynovitis: a clinical study of 544 cases in industry. *Br. J. Industr. Med.*, **8**, 150–8.

Tillaux, P. (1892) *Traité d'anatomie topographique. Avec applications à la chirurgie*, ed. 7. Asselin et Houzeau, Paris.

Travell, J., Rinzler, S. and Herman, M. (1942) Pain and disability of the shoulder and arm, treatment by intramuscular infiltration with procaine hydrochloride. *JAMA*, **120**(6), 417–22.

Travell, J.G. and Simons, D.G. (1983) *The Trigger Point Manual*. Williams & Wilkins, Baltimore, Md.

Troell, A. (1918) Uber die sogenannte tendovaginitis crepitans. *Dtsch. Z. Chir.*, **143**, 125–62.

Velpeau, A. (1825) Anatomie des regions. Traite d'anatomie chirurgicale, vol. 1. Crevot, Paris, pp. 402–15.

Wall, P.D. (1986) Causes of intractable pain. *Hospital Update*, December, pp. 969–74.

Wall, P.D. (1991) Neuropathic pain and injured nerve: central mechanisms. *Br. Med. Bull.*, **47**(3), 631–43.

Wigley, R.D., Turner, W.E.D., Blake, B.L., Darby, F.W., McInnes, R. and Harding, P. (1992) Occupational overuse syndrome. Treatment and rehabilitation: a practitioner's guide. Occupational Safety and Health Service, Department of Labour, Wellington, NZ.

Woolf, C.J. (1991) Generation of acute pain: central mechanisms. *Br. Med. Bull.*, **47**(3), 523–33.

2

Concepts and controversies

During the past century of advance the art of medicine has not kept pace with the science of disease.
Waddell et al. (1984)

Apologia

My apologies are offered to those readers who have always thought (as I used to think) that the aetiology of common conditions such as lateral and medial epicondylitis is relatively clear-cut. During my years in general practice, and in my early years in specialist practice, there seemed little doubt (as stated by Cyriax many years previously) that lateral epicondylitis and medial epicondylitis resulted from overuse of the common extensors or common flexors of the wrist and hand. Indeed, I retain the opinion that in the majority of cases the aetiology is relatively clearly defined. However, there are two principal reasons to persuade one to think otherwise.

Some years ago I was astonished to discover a body of medical opinion that views these conditions affecting the epicondylar entheses as 'constitutional', not caused by repetitive physical activities wherever they might take place, but arising perhaps from malign providence. In support of this view it is stated that epidemiological evidence for a causal relationship with work from properly controlled studies is scanty (Viikari-Juntura, 1984). However, a counterbalancing argument is that there is more substantive evidence for an association between lateral epicondylitis and sport such as tennis in which repetitive grasping (of a racquet) is an inherent characteristic. Enthesopathies elsewhere (for example, patellar tendinitis and

adductor longus tendinitis) are also considered to be a result of overuse. Reflecting on causation, the reader may appreciate the distinction between sports, recreational and domestic activities on the one hand, and work (with its connotation of employer liability) on the other. One needs to take account of the potential confounding dimensions given to the problems of diagnosis, management and prognosis by the issues of causation and liability.

As a consequence of the expansion of my clinical practice to include an increasing number of cases of *refractory* musculoskeletal disorders, irrespective of causation but commonly work-related, it has become apparent to me that diffuse pain around the elbow and in the forearm, sometimes bilateral, is a feature of the regional pain syndrome referred to in this text as type 2 WRULD (work-related upper limb disorder). In this condition there is persistent widespread pain and hyperalgesia in the neck, pectoral girdle and upper limb. An **awareness** of the possibility of type 2 WRULD is a prerequisite to a correct diagnosis in cases of elbow pain. The importance of a specific diagnosis as opposed to a nominal diagnosis of 'elbow pain' cannot be overstressed, particularly as the therapeutic strategies in the management of enthesopathies and type 2 WRULD are quite different. The prognosis is vastly different. The concept of type 2 WRULD is explored further in subsequent chapters.

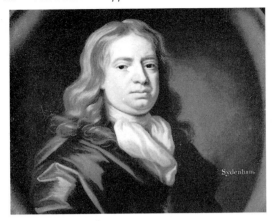

Figure 2.1 Thomas Sydenham (1624–89) developed the prototype of the disease–illness model

The disease–illness model

An explanation for the emergence of the present-day controversies surrounding the aetiology of work-related upper limb disorders is difficult without an historical review of medical epistemology – the study of the manner in which medical knowledge has been constructed and utilized.

Twentieth-century medicine has been based (comfortably) upon the **disease–illness** model, the prototype of which was developed by Thomas Sydenham (1624–89) (Figure 2.1). Sydenham, who was often described as the 'English Hippocrates', classified disease as acute (caused by God) and chronic (caused by Man). He recognized the need for the further classification of diseases in general into separate disease entities or 'morbid species' (thereby, incidentally, inaugurating the science of nosology).

Of relevance to the study of work-related upper limb disorders, Sydenham emphasized the importance of establishing the aetiology of disease. He took a nihilistic approach to the contemporary theoretical sciences, promulgating positivism at the expense of fatalism. His most important contribution was to recognize the need to examine patients carefully, to make a specific diagnosis rather than refer to symptom complexes (or syndromes – as we would now call them) and to treat accordingly. I suspect that Sydenham would have eschewed the late-twentieth-century tendency to engage in tautological concepts such as the

hypothesis that tender muscle is the intrinsic component of the myofascial pain syndrome (which is defined as a condition characterized by referred pain from trigger points in muscles).

In relation to upper limb pain, Sydenham's basic disease–illness paradigm was redefined over the next two centuries to the extent that the 'illness' – the manifestations of the disease process affecting the soft tissues and nerves – was studied in some considerable detail by the great physicians and neurologists (such as Poore and Gowers) at the end of the nineteenth century. Their observations of the illness – the demeanour of those patients afflicted by (what Gowers termed as) 'occupational neuroses' – provided the means whereby diverse pathophysiological interpretations could be applied to the disease process (Poore, 1878; Gowers, 1892). For instance, whilst favouring a central (nervous system) origin for upper limb symptoms, Gowers placed considerable weight on the concept of vulnerability or susceptibility: anything that 'lowers the tone of the nervous system may doubtless act as a predisposing cause'.

Pain perception

Aristotle (384–322 BC) (Figure 2.2) distilled the vision of the Ancient Greek philosophers regarding sensory phenomena into his theory of the five senses: vision, hearing, taste, smell and touch. He considered pain to be an increased sensitivity of every sensation, particularly touch, and pain perception to be felt in the heart. The Aristotelian concept of pain as an affective manifestation – a 'passion of the soul' felt in the heart – prevailed for well over two millennia despite the conviction of his successors such as Herophilus and Erasistratus that the centre of sensation was located in the brain, and the views of Galen (AD 131–200), who established the anatomy of the central and autonomic nervous systems, and more 'recently' of René Descartes (1596–1650) (Figure 2.3), who further defined the concept of the skin–nerve–brain pain pathway.

Gradually, throughout the latter half of the nineteenth century, a specificity theory of pain gained ascendency over a summation theory. In the latter, stimulus intensity and central

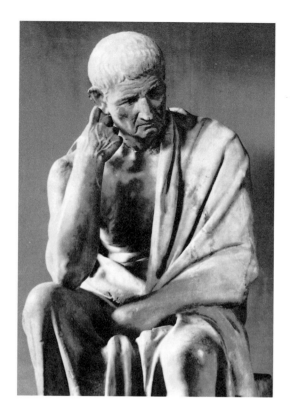

Figure 2.2 Aristotle (384–322 BC) considered that pain perception – a 'passion of the soul' – was felt in the heart

twentieth century progressed, scientific evidence began to suggest that pain was determined by a larger number of physiological and psychological variables.

The seminal work of Melzack and Wall (1965) on the **gate control theory** of pain provided the physiological basis for an explanation of the observed pain phenomena and the affective and cognitive aspects of pain. The transmission of afferent nerve impulses was considered to be modulated at spinal dorsal horn level by a gating mechanism. Several interacting neural systems, including those from higher centres ('beyond the gate') have an excitatory or inhibitory function at the gate. When neural transmission reaches a critical level, and the gate is opened, a complex pattern of responses results in the experience and manifestation of pain.

Almost at a stroke the gate control theory replaced the previously held Cartesian mind–body dichotomy theory and, as a result, prompted the expansion of the holistic view of medicine that had been gaining ground. Additionally, it validated the development of a different clinical approach to illness that was

summation were the critical determinants of pain. In the **specificity theory** pain was a specific sensation with its own sensory apparatus independent of touch and other senses: inherent in the concept of specificity was a specific response to a specific stimulus (Bonica, 1990). It is apparent that by the beginning of the twentieth century (and for a considerable time thereafter), medical opinions had become influenced strongly by the concept of the mind–body dichotomy of Descartes and the Cartesian view of pain as a straightforward response to a physical stimulus.

To account for the known psychological factors that influence pain, the concept of the **duality of pain** was proposed (and subsequently refined in the period around the middle of the twentieth century by Hardy *et al.*, 1952): the distinct features were neurophysiological (perception of pain) and psychophysiological (reaction to pain). However, as the

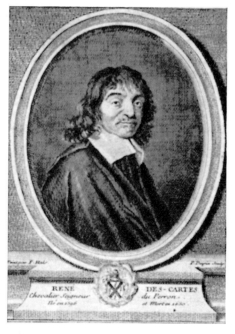

Figure 2.3 René Descartes (1596–1650) refined the concept of the skin–nerve–brain pain pathway, the precursor of the concept of the duality of pain

being formulated in the behavioural sciences. The recent development of the concept of **chronic pain** (in which the pain itself becomes the disease rather than being a symptom of disease) has led to further progress in the understanding of regional pain syndromes. This book further explores this concept.

A biopsychosocial concept of illness

Over tne past twenty years the disease–illness model in locomotor medicine has been further refined, at least as applied to back pain, by Waddell (1987). Basing his operational model for clinical practice on Loeser's biopsychosocial concept of illness (Loeser and Fordyce, 1983) (Figure 2.4*a*), the Glasgow illness model emerged (Figure 2.4*b*), emphasizing the outward expression of physical disease as illness behaviour (Waddell *et al.*, 1984). The manifestations of a disease process – the functional disability, distress and chronic illness behaviour – were distinguished from the pathoanatomical and pathophysiological aspects of the disease process itself.

Although distress and illness behaviour (for instance, anxiety and increased body awareness) are 'secondary to' the physical disorder, Waddell stated that they may be influenced in severity or longevity by the success or failure of treatment, and also by unrelated stresses. Waddell advised that 'we must distinguish pain from disability, the symptoms and signs of distress and illness behaviour from those of physical disease, and nominal from substantive diagnoses'. Although referring primarily to back pain, his observations may equally well be transposed to the concept of pain in the neck and arm.

Psychosocial factors are often critical to the prognosis for back pain (Figure 2.5). Outcome of treatment depends on these factors, particularly coping strategies, to a considerably greater extent than conventional clinical information (Burton *et al.*, 1995).

Illness behaviour

The stimulus provided by Waddell has led to much attention being directed to the behavioural responses of patients to chronic musculoskeletal conditions in general. The increasing

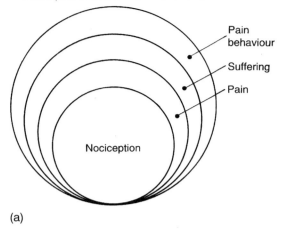

A conceptual model of pain (Loeser)

Pain behaviour
Suffering
Pain
Nociception

(a)

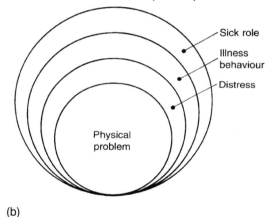

A clinical model of illness (Waddell)

Sick role
Illness behaviour
Distress
Physical problem

(b)

Figure 2.4 Waddell based the Glasgow illness model (*b*) on Loeser's concept of illness (*a*)

(medical) awareness of the significance of illness behaviour (and, as a consequence, the behavioural cognitive-behavioural management strategies for those who manifest abnormal illness behaviour) has enabled the concept of maladaptation by patients with chronic pain to psychosocial stresses to be distinguished from the 'accident neurosis' concept of the neurologist Henry Miller (1961).

Although Miller, an eminent neurologist, chose to use the term 'accident neurosis' rather than 'compensation neurosis' or 'litigation neurosis' as (he conceded that) the latter terms prejudged the issue, he was in little

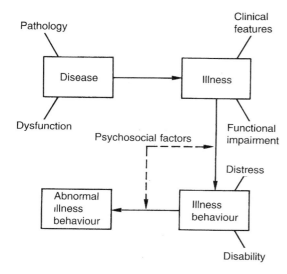

Figure 2.5 Psychosocial factors have a critical role in the development of illness behaviour

doubt that the condition 'is not encountered' where the hope of financial gain does not exist. He came to this conclusion following the examination of 200 cases of 'head injury' referred to him for medicolegal reporting in the 1950s. Interestingly, the behaviour of the patients at his examination, their steadfast attitude of 'martyred gloom', and their unshakeable conviction of unfitness for work, is similar to a (minority) subgroup of litigants in cases of work-related upper limb disorders (WRULDs).

In my experience, however, the majority of patients with a WRULD who proceed to litigation do not grossly dramatize their symptoms, and do not exhibit the extreme behaviour responses described by Miller. In the light of recent research on neuropathic pain and its potential behavioural consequences, Miller's interpretations of the cause of distress and the adoption of the sick role in patients with no physical signs of 'organic disease' look increasingly dated.

Abnormal illness behaviour

The concept of abnormal illness behaviour (AIB) and its relationship to real or perceived somatic disturbances was introduced by Pilowsky (1969). In an attempt to clarify such vague syndromes as 'functional overlay' (which was a fashionable term and concept during my medical training in the early 1960s, and is still used today), Pilowsky (1978) classified abnormal illness behaviours into those that were somatically focused and those that were psychologically focused. He defined AIB as 'the persistence of an *inappropriate* or *maladaptive* mode of perceiving, evaluating and acting in relation to one's state of health' (my italics).

The application of abnormal ('inappropriate') illness behaviour (AIB) to patients with musculoskeletal pain was made by Waddell, according to whom patients with 'magnified' or 'inappropriate' illness behaviour locate their pain and dysaesthesiae in a widespread fashion, using emotive terms; a pain diagram is deemed to be a useful tool in this assessment. He considered that 'inappropriate' physical signs include widespread 'non-anatomic' tenderness and specific tests for 'non-disease'. These tests include the provocation of low back pain on axial loading of the spine and on simulated spinal rotation (Waddell *et al.*, 1984; Waddell, 1987).

However, Waddell's interpretation of the 'inappropriateness' of some of the symptoms and signs is very questionable in the context of our present state of knowledge of neuroplasticity. For instance, 'superficial, widespread, non-anatomical tenderness' may more easily be explained as allodynia and secondary hyperalgesia (a neurogenic concept indicating hypersensitivity of the nervous system as a response to soft tissue injury, see Chapter 3) than as a sign of inappropriate illness behaviour. A further concern is that it is not clear whether Waddell gave due (or any) credence to the role of somatic (spinal) dysfunction in back pain. Nevertheless, Waddell emphasized the role of illness behaviour and distress in the expression of musculoskeletal problems – a sea-change in medical attitudes.

Affirmation of the validity of the concept of distress in patients with musculoskeletal pain has come from the disciplines of pain relief (Tyrer, 1986) and rheumatology (Helliwell, 1992). Tyrer refers to 'learned pain behaviour' and emphasizes that this may occur in patients with physical injury: 'it is not synonymous with non-organic pain'. Helliwell states that 'the psychological distress indicated by Waddell's non-organic signs does not mean the patient is malingering but that there

A neuropathic model of pain (Hutson)

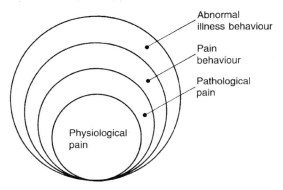

Figure 2.6 A model of pain that acknowledges the roles of nervous system sensitization and abnormal illness behaviour

are non-physical factors which need to be dealt with in order to effect a successful outcome'. The behavioural expression of pain that is demonstrated in Figure 2.6 acknowledges the intimate relationship with neurosensitization.

Factors which may encourage maladaptive behaviour include the advice to rest until pain has *fully* resolved, loss of functional independence, loss of work, a solicitous and overprotective family which encourages dependence, and the vain pursuit of further diagnosis and treatment (Williams *et al.*, 1993). Poor relationships at work, the litigation process, and substandard medical expertise (particularly with respect to the lack of recognition and management of chronic pain) are further important stressors. The iatrogenic component is regrettable but commonly present.

Joyce Williams (1989) described the behavioural characteristics of more than 500 patients with back pain referred by doctors who could 'do nothing more for them'. After labelling the condition 'the thick file syndrome' initially, it became apparent to Williams and her co-workers that the exaggerated pain and illness behaviours adopted by patients were a result of distress. As abnormal illness behaviour is also observed in a subgroup of patients with work-related neck and arm pain, most commonly those with type 2 WRULD, some of the more salient features are listed below. It is important to realize that AIB should only be diagnosed when a significant number (four to six or more) of features are present.

- Lack of eye contact.
- Lack of spontaneous gestures.
- Lack of affect; depressed facies.
- Overt badges of invalidism (Figure 2.7) – cervical collars; lumbar supports (may be carried); walking sticks; wheelchairs.
- Excessively slow, deliberate movements.
- Initial freezing and repetitive starts.
- Apparent excessive effort and difficulty in ordinary activities such as dressing/undressing.
- Frequent pain gestures (to indicate suffering) – grimacing; holding/touching affected area; excessively protective; vocalization ('phew' or similar sounds).
- Abnormal posture, gait or movement pattern – antalgic position of upper limb; wide-based gait; no arm swing.
- Abnormal balance; staggering.
- Illness postures: feeling of faintness or dizziness.

Williams concedes that abnormal behaviour may result from the anticipation of financial gain or compensation of some type. When such patients were excluded from rehabilitation treatment in the 'School for Bravery' approach, 80% of patients with (AIB and) chronic pain were converted from a state of illness behaviour to wellness. When patients anticipating financial gain were included, the likelihood of success dropped to 20%.

Psychogenic concepts

It is generally recognized that chronic pain is associated with depression. The causal relationship is unclear, however, and has led to much debate. Other psychological disturbances such as early childhood deprivation (including abandonment, abuse and emotional isolation), marital and family difficulties, and personality disorder have also been cited as primary contributors to (psychogenic) chronic pain. The outcome of spinal surgery has been shown to be dependent on abandonment and abuse in a prospective study (Schofferman *et al.*, 1992).

Gamsa (1990) questioned the adequacy of methodology in many past studies, and compared a substantive number of chronic pain

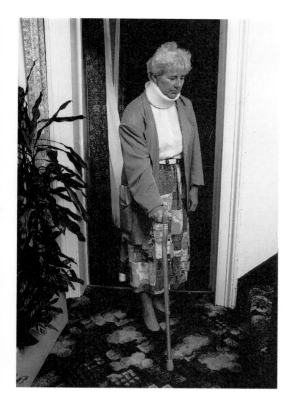

Figure 2.7 Overt badges of invalidism: a cervical collar, a walking stick and a lumbar corset stuffed into the jacket pocket

sufferers with a control group when explaining the relationship between psychological factors and pain. She concluded that the emotional disturbance is more likely to be a consequence than a cause of chronic pain.

Whilst it is likely that some (probably a minority of) patients with refractory upper limb disorders suffer from psychogenic pain, it is unwise to invoke a psychogenic diagnosis simply on the basis of no demonstrable organic disease. It could be argued that the readiness with which some doctors diagnose 'RSI' on flimsy evidence (Awerbuch, 1986) is matched by the enthusiasm by others for 'non-disease' or 'somatization' in patients whose pain is 'apparently discordant with discernible abnormalities' (Awerbuch, 1995).

The central theme of non-disease and somatization is that 'failure to recognize that pain is a symptom which does not necessarily indicate physical injury or disease could lead to misdiagnosis, particularly if the diagnosis is based on subjective rather than objective criteria'. Somatizing patients are considered to be particularly receptive to diagnoses which carry the flavour of organicity and authenticity ('now I know it's not in my head'). The tactile findings of allodynia, hyperalgesia, and sudomotor changes are often ignored or deprecated, and their acknowledgement by clinicians specializing in manual therapy (such as musculoskeletal physicians, osteopaths and chiropractors) is sometimes criticized as manifesting a lack of clinical objectivity.

There appear to be two major dangers in the diagnosis of somatization. First, the assumption that somatization (or the twinned nihilistic concept of non-disease) equates with abnormal illness behaviour. Although traditional explanations for somatization, including hysteria and hypochondriasis, have been criticized as loose and pejorative (Murphy, 1989), the modern concept (at least in the UK) of somatization as a patient's 'misattribution' of bodily symptoms to organic disease is not identical to a patient's maladaptive responses to pain (as is the situation with AIB). **Somatic symptoms, whether psychogenic or organic, should be distinguished from the behavioural responses to these symptoms**.

Secondly, and the crux of this apparent paradox of discordance on examination, is the basis on which 'no discernible abnormalities' is founded. Doctors who have received inadequate (or 'no') training in basic musculoskeletal medicine, and therefore have not developed the clinical expertise required to detect (and consequently to interpret) the signs of musculoskeletal dysfunction (for instance, loss of joint play in spinal joints), and neural dysfunction (for instance, altered responses to tactile and mechanoprovocative tests), are at a substantial disadvantage. Furthermore, the reliance by psychiatrists and psychologists (for instance, Lucire, 1986) upon the diagnosis of 'non-(organic) disease' by their medical colleagues who are responsible for their patients' musculoskeletal examination makes them vulnerable to misattribution of somatic symptoms to psychological syndromes.

Merskey (1984) warned against sloppy psychological labelling which has the potential to deny patients appropriate physical treatment. A psychogenic diagnosis should be substantiated by sound psychiatric evidence in the same manner in which a diagnosis of neuromusculoskeletal dysfunction is made. Wall (1994) advised that 'the contemporary custom of assigning the cause of pain either to peripheral pathology or to mental pathology is too simple because it ignores the subtle dynamic properties of peripheral tissue and of the nervous system'.

Myofascial pain

The concept of the myofascial pain syndrome (MPS) has been developed by Travell and Simons. The disorder is described as a regional muscle pain disorder that is characterized by localized muscle tenderness and pain, the pathognomonic feature of which is the myofascial trigger point (commonly referred to as a TP or TrP). A myofascial trigger point is defined as 'a hyperirritable spot, usually within a taut band of skeletal muscle or in the muscle's fascia, that is painful on compression and that can give rise to characteristic referred pain, tenderness and autonomic phenomena' (Travell and Simons, 1983). The taut band represents an area of muscle tension and shortening. A local twitch response from the taut band manifests clinically as the 'jump sign' in which the patient reacts by grimacing or vocalizing their pain on palpation of the trigger point. Treatment is directed towards 'inactivation' of the relevant trigger point by dry needling, local anaesthetic injections, deep ischaemic compression, or superficial cold applications, any of which should be followed by stretching. Spread and chronicity are explained by the activation of latent, secondary or satellite trigger points.

In the context of upper limb pain, the concept of myofascial pain that is attributable to areas of primary hyperalgesia has been criticized by Quintner and Cohen (1994). They consider that the propositions 'MPS (myofascial pain syndrome) is a regional pain syndrome associated with dysfunction of one or more muscles – trigger points, that have a discrete reference zone of pain' and 'trigger points are the primary feature of the myofascial pain syndrome' constitute a circular and tautological argument: the definition of the syndrome incorporates the preferred hypothesis of causation, and by virtue of its form the proposition must always be true. Indeed,

the sheer number of syndromes ascribed to the myofascial pain concept must call into question its validity (Campbell, 1989).

Although accepted as an entity, the trigger point lacks clinical reliability. Latent, 'metastasizing' and secondary trigger points lack supporting evidence. There is no support for the myofascial pain syndrome from animal experimental models, from human muscle injuries, or from histological studies. Furthermore, taut bands and muscle twitch responses are as common in healthy volunteers as in myofascial pain syndrome and fibromyalgia syndrome (Wolfe, 1992). By contrast, Quintner and Cohen suggest that the phenomenon of the trigger point, on which depends the theory of the myofascial pain syndrome, is better understood as a region of secondary hyperalgesia of peripheral nerve origin.

A further explanation for the persistence of symptoms and tender points in the upper limb in regional pain syndromes is referred pain from the neck. Smythe (1994) has expanded upon this bedrock of osteopathic principles by defining patterns of tenderness at specific sites in the neck, pectoral girdle and upper limb when mechanically acting segmental factors are operative at either the C5–6 or the C6–7 levels (see Cervical Spinal Lesions, Chapter 5). Appropriate nocturnal support, mechanical in the form of a specially shaped pillow, and postural by the adoption of the fetal position, are his recommended treatment strategies.

Whatever the originating factor, trigger points show features of sympathetic nervous activity, and maintenance of the trigger point appears to depend on this activity (Hubbard and Berkoff, 1993).

It is generally recognized that the absence of epidemiological data with respect to myofascial pain hinders the more widespread acceptance by the medical profession of the concept of chronic pain from muscles. Undoubtedly, the reliance upon *palpation* of muscle hypertonus gives rise to poor inter-observer reliability. However, in a reflective and balanced view on myofascial pain, Hancock (1995) suggests that 'the concept of the myofascial trigger point should be subsumed into a wider neurophysiological understanding of the meaning of muscle tenderness, rather than regarded as a local mechanical-ischaemic pathophysiological disturbance'.

In my opinion, **the concept of secondary hyperalgesia reconciles satisfactorily the clinical finding of muscle tenderness** (thereby offering an explanation for pain experienced in conditions such as type 2 WRULD, and the chronic whiplash syndrome).

Adverse neural tension

The concept of neural tension in the upper limb was developed by Elvey in Australia (1986). His brachial plexus tension test (BPTT) was based on cadaveric studies in which mobility and tension of cervical nerve roots and their investing dural sheaths were demonstrated with arm movements; maximal responses were noted at C5 and C6. Elvey's brachial plexus tension test, sometimes described as 'the straight leg raise of the arm', was designed to place the neural tissues (including the cervical nerve roots, brachial plexus and peripheral nerves) under maximum tension (see also Chapter 7). The purpose of the test was to differentiate neural tension from tension of the soft tissues (the muscles, bursae and joint capsules in the neck and shoulder region).

It has been noted by many observers, particularly the physiotherapy profession, that many patients with the regional pain syndrome referred to as type 2 WRULD in this text exhibit positive signs of adverse neural tension on careful examination. A somewhat simplistic explanation of this observation is that the diffuse symptoms and tender points in the upper limb are the result of primary nerve root compression or irritation. Although this may accurately represent the situation in some patients, the probability is that rather more complicated neurophysiological mechanisms are involved in many cases, not least the likelihood of increased mechanosensitivity as part of a neuropathic process. Accordingly, the term 'neurodynamic testing' has been introduced (Shacklock, 1995) in recognition of the role of both mechanical and physiological mechanisms in the 'tension tests'.

The natural consequence of the concept of abnormal neurodynamics is that mechanical mobilization of the neural tissues may have a practical therapeutic application by influencing pain physiology in a useful way. Although the exact mechanism(s) of the response of tissues to mobilization and manipulation have not been fully evaluated, neural mobilization is seen by some physiotherapists as a useful addition to their therapeutic armamentarium.

For *aficionados*, Butler (1991) has described a series of tension tests with a selective bias for the median, radial and ulnar nerves. As a screening test, however, the brachial plexus tension test described by Elvey remains in common usage.

Fatalism and non-intervention

Within the past decade, the aetiology, diagnosis and management of work-related disorders has been obfuscated by the concept of fatalism. This proposes that most of the musculoskeletal disorders affecting the upper limb that are discussed in this book arise from 'constitutional' causes, whatever they might be. The observation that we are all afflicted at some time or another by symptoms such as backache or arm ache confirms their ubiquity and inevitability. Accordingly, runs the argument, although arm pain may be manifest at work, there is no causal relationship with work activities.

The chronicity of some conditions is explained by the failure of coping skills when the sufferer is confronted by overwhelming psychosocial changes (Hadler, 1993). Consequently, inappropriate diagnostic labelling by the physician provides the basis for the adoption by the patient (unwittingly possibly) of the *illness of work incapacity* and/or the adoption of the *role of litigant*.

The fatalistic attitude with respect to the universality and inevitability of musculoskeletal symptoms, and the moralistic view with respect to the claimed pivotal role of the medical profession in the conversion of indisposition to disability, create an undesirable smoke-screen. Clinical assessments and legal judgments should be based on the singular factors pertaining to a particular case. I suspect that, should a comprehensive musculoskeletal examination be directed towards the detection of the manifestations of spinal dysfunction and neural plasticity as well as the overt expressions of peripheral pathology, there would be fewer syndromic diagnoses such as 'periarthritis' and 'neck pain' and fewer disgruntled patients.

The exclusion of dysfunction of the soft tissues and neural systems from the differential diagnosis of arm pain reduces *ipso facto* the considered therapeutic options. Hence, the espousal of the concept of management by non-intervention to avoid the use of 'unproven remedies' is typified by Hadler's views on spinal manipulation for back pain: 'I, personally, neither advise nor perform this manoeuvre; the benefit is small and the procedure itself is *personally repugnant*' (Hadler, 1993, p. 10; my italics). In an era of increasing enlightenment with respect to tissue plasticity in the pathogenesis of many musculoskeletal disorders (including the concepts of reversible spinal joint dysfunction and neural irritation arising at spinal level), it is difficult to reconcile non-interventionism with the use by doctors and therapists with appropriate training of a spectrum of manual techniques, including manipulation, to moderate soft tissue dysfunction.

Epistemological flaws

Regrettably, the concepts of *soft tissue plasticity* and *joint dysfunction*, both axial and peripheral, have been slow to gain acceptance in mainstream medicine. As a result, late twentieth-century medical diagnoses continue to be predicated upon gross morphological and histochemical pathology that have developed over the previous two hundred years. However, strict adherence to the disease–illness model and denial of the concept of distress (or 'dis-ease') is to be deplored. The adoption of Cartesian dualism, whereby, in the absence of firm evidence of relevant pathology, patients' complaints are considered to be fanciful, or a mental aberration, is epistemologically unsound.

The 'structuralist' demand for an identifiable organic basis (in the form of histopathological evidence) of tissue disease or dystrophy in overuse conditions of the upper limb (Barton *et al.*, 1992; Hadler, 1985; Ireland, 1988) is often reinforced by a demand by the protagonists of evidence-based medicine for *absolute* epidemiological evidence (from randomized controlled trials) to establish the credibility of work-relatedness in patients suffering from conditions such as de Quervain's tenovaginitis. These criteria are separate issues, however. The purist concept of detectable peripheral pathology as the most credible basis for regional pain syndromes is becoming increasingly dated with the discovery of the cascade of changes in the central nervous system after peripheral pathology has disappeared (Wall, 1994).

Personal bias leads quickly to entrenched misconceptions. Reflective views at the time of the Australian 'epidemic' in the 1980s, such as those of Ferguson (1987) – 'with hindsight, the gigantic and costly Australian epidemic called "repetition strain injury" ("RSI") can be seen as a complex psychosocial phenomenon with elements of mass hysteria, that were superimposed on a basis of widespread discomfort, fatigue and morbidity' – were matched by the pejorative opinions of Awerbuch and others. Even the views of Brooks (1989) – 'the majority of patients with chronic pain have only that' – are hardly compatible with a sympathetic attitude to patients' upper limb problems in the 1990s. The philosophy of non-disease is unhelpful and Nelsonian; the lack of a specific diagnosis should not automatically imply the presence of somatization. Pilowsky (1985) identified the possibility of medical bias by coining the phrase 'malingerophobia' to describe a disease of doctors who are so frightened of compensating malingerers that they are prepared to penalize the deserving majority.

Contributory factors to faulty epistemology are the failure to conduct an adequate musculoskeletal examination (which should include a *functional* assessment of the spinal and peripheral joints, the muscles and tendons of the upper limb and the central and autonomic nervous systems) and the more fundamental failure to grasp that **somatic dysfunction** – a disturbance of spinal function that is not demonstrable by contemporary scientific investigative techniques – or **neuropathia** can account for muscle tenderness and referred pain and dysaesthesia in the upper limb.

The difficulties experienced by orthopaedists when assessing the soft tissues of the cervical spine have been summarized by Gargan (1995): '*Hard physical signs* [my italics] are rare following whiplash, and many orthopaedic colleagues are uncomfortable with the concept of a disease model that does not have such signs as a predominant feature.' Recognition of the positive attributes of the orthodox orthopaedic approach to major structural problems of the spine is tempered by its conceptual and practical shortcomings in soft tissue disturbances. The introduction during orthopaedic training of tuition in musculoskeletal medical techniques for the detection of joint dysfunction should partially overcome this deficit.

Epidemiological flaws

Studies of many musculoskeletal conditions, particularly dysfunctional states in which there is no consistent histopathology, face severe methodological problems. Attributing causation from cross-sectional surveys and other types of studies is hazardous; case-control studies are notoriously prone to bias, and there have been few double-blinded random case-controlled trials on the efficacy of treatments.

There is often little agreement on the appropriate clinical tests for a specific condition, and therefore little prospect of standardization of diagnosis. In some conditions such as rotator cuff tendinitis, there appears to be general acceptance of isometric contraction pain (described by Cyriax, 1969) as the principal diagnostic criterion; in other conditions in which hyperalgesia is a feature, inter-observer error is undoubtedly high (Wolfe *et al.*, 1992). The usefulness of investigations such as magnetic resonance imaging (MRI) is limited: this is an expensive procedure and of little value in dysfunctional conditions. Although electrodiagnosis is often upheld as the most reliable indicator of nerve entrapment, it may yield negative results in the early stages of nerve compression syndromes.

Outcome measures following intervention are equally fraught with problems. Most assessments rely on the measurement of pain, a wholly subjective phenomenon for which the visual analogue scale is most frequently used despite its obvious drawbacks. In pain augmentation states the use of devices to standardize noxious stimuli in order to make partially objective measurements of the pain perception threshold or the pain tolerance threshold is largely confined to research programmes.

In practice, several sources of information on work-related disorders are available: 'common' knowledge, insurance and occupational health data, cross-sectional surveys, longitudinal studies of cohorts and case-control studies (Bjelle, 1989). Longitudinal studies are particularly important, but are time-consuming and expensive. Selection bias is often a problem unless the methodology is strictly controlled, and the study numbers are sufficiently large.

On a more positive note, meaningful research into soft tissue disorders is possible and indeed is being carried out. Vital to its success is the definition of appropriate *diagnostic, selection and outcome criteria*.

'Proof' is not always easy to come by in the field of musculoskeletal disorders. Writing on the credibility of a hypothesis, Karl Popper (1959; see also Popper, 1972) advised that greater emphasis should be placed upon the rejection of potentially falsifiable evidence rather than upon the acquisition of positive supportive evidence. This scientific philosophy is particularly relevant to musculoskeletal medicine. When supported by multi-observer empirical findings, reasonable hypotheses should be considered with due weight and not rejected unless there is sound evidence to the contrary.

Summary

Inappropriate diagnoses frequently result from inadequate clinical expertise, including the failure by the physician to recognize distress or the sense of grievance that is often associated with the symptoms of soft tissue or neural 'disease' in patients with upper limb disorders. A common complaint from a 'constitutionalist' (one who believes that the vast majority of upper limb syndromes are constitutional in origin) is that medical practitioners who propose work-relatedness too readily may encourage or even cause this feeling of grievance, particularly in a potential litigant. Regrettably, the obverse is usually true – that is, the grievance more often results from a lack of medical acumen, a combination of poor examining skills and insufficient understanding of the aetiological factors associated with the condition and the reason for the patient's distress. Of course, some of these cases are difficult to treat successfully, but medical intransigence is often to blame for chronicity.

Iatrogenic disease is only too common in cases coming to medicolegal contest – not so much as a consequence of the 'abnormal diagnostic behaviour' of those medical practitioners perceived by Awerbuch (1986) to be too easily misled into diagnosing RSI, but as a result of the lack of vision of others.

We should recognize the role played by the following:

- Neuroplasticity.
- Decompensation (loss of adaptation) of the musculotendinous and articular structures ('disease' according to the disease–illness model) and consequential loss of function.
- The pathophysiological state of neuropathia (a 'disease' of pain production) and the intimately associated behavioural responses of the patient ('distress'), the combination of the two giving rise to loss of functional independence.
- Abnormal illness behaviour (AIB) which often has a strong iatrogenic component in its aetiology as well as diverse psychosocial associations.

We should eschew:

- Primary psychogenic labels – unless appropriate efforts (if necessary, including an examination by a musculoskeletal physician) have been made to exclude nerve, muscle, tendon and joint **dysfunction**.
- A fatalistic approach. The average person living in the Western hemisphere at the end of the twentieth century simply does not have the patience to accept the therapeutic philosophy of non-intervention ('and society has learnt to turn to science rather than to philosophy for the solution to its predicaments, much to its peril', Hadler, 1993).
- The sophistry inherent in the arrogant dismissal of the concepts of musculoskeletal dysfunction and/or neuropathia without due consideration.

References

Awerbuch, M. (1986) RSI. *Med. J. Aust.*, **145**, 362–3.

Awerbuch, M. (1995) Different concepts of chronic musculoskeletal pain. *Ann. Rheumat. Dis.*, **54**, 331–2.

Barton, N.J., Hooper, G., Noble, J. and Steel, W.M. (1992) Occupational cause of disorders in the upper limb. *Br. Med. J.*, **304**, 309–11.

Bjelle, A. (1989) Epidemiology of shoulder problems. *Baillière's Clinical Rheumatology*, **3**(3), 437–51.

Bonica, J.J. (1990) *Management of Pain*, vol. 1, 2nd edn. Lea and Febiger, Philadelphia, pp. 2–17.

Brooks, P. (1989) RSI – regional pain syndrome: the importance of nomenclature. *Br. J. Rheumatol.*, **28**, 180–2.

Burton, A.K., Tillotson, K.M., Main, C.J. and Hollis, S. (1995) Psychosocial predictors of outcome in acute and subchronic low back trouble. *Spine*, **20**(6), 722–8.

Butler, D.S. (1991) Tension testing – the upper limbs. In: *Mobilization of the Nervous System*, Churchill Livingstone, Melbourne, pp. 147–60.

Campbell, S.M. (1989) Regional myofascial pain syndromes. *Rheumatol. Dis. Clin. North Am.*, **15**(1), 31–44.

Cyriax, J.H. (1969) *Textbook of Orthopaedic Medicine: Diagnosis of Soft-tissue Lesions*, 5th edn. Baillière, Tindall, Cassell, London.

Elvey, R.L. (1986) Treatment of arm pain associated with abnormal brachial plexus tension. *Aust. J. Physiotherapy*, **32**, 224–9.

Ferguson D. (1987) RSI: putting the epidemic to rest. *Med. J. Aust.* **147**, 213–14.

Gamsa, A. (1990) Is emotional disturbance a precipitator or a consequence of chronic pain? *Pain*, **42**, 183–95.

Gargan, M.F. (1995) What is the evidence for an organic lesion in whiplash injury? *J. Psychosomat. Res.*, **39**(6), 777–81.

Gowers, W.R. (1892) *A Manual of Diseases of the Nervous System*, vol. 2. Churchill, London, pp. 656–76; 710–30.

Hadler, N.M. (1985) Illness in the workplace: the challenge of musculoskeletal symptoms. *J. Hand Surg.*, **10A**(4), 451–6.

Hadler, N.M. (1993) *Occupational Musculoskeletal Disorders*. Raven Press, New York.

Hancock, J. (1995) Comments on Barnsley *et al.* [Barnsley *et al.* (1994) Whiplash injury. *Pain*, **58**, 283–307]. *Pain*, 61, 487–95.

Hardy, J.D., Wolff, H.G. and Goodell, H. (1952) *Pain Sensations and Reactions*. Williams and Wilkins, Baltimore.

Helliwell, P.S. (1992) Occupational rheumatology: are we using the wrong model? *Br. J. Rheumatol.*, **31**, 73–6.

Hubbard, D.R. and Berkoff, G.M. (1993) Myofascial trigger points show spontaneous needle EMG activity. *Spine*, **18**, 1803–7.

Ireland, D.C.R. (1988) Psychological and physical aspects of occupational arm pain. *J. Hand Surg.*, **13B**(1), 5–10.

Loeser, J.D. and Fordyce, W.E. (1983) Chronic pain. In: *Behavioural Science in the Practice of Medicine* (eds J.E. Carr and H.A. Dengerink, Elsevier, New York.

Lucire, Y. (1986) Neurosis in the workplace. *Med. J. Aust.*, **145**, 323–7.

Melzack, R. and Wall, P.D. (1965) Pain mechanisms: a new theory. *Science*, **150**, 971–9.

Merskey, H. (1984). Symptoms that depress the doctor: too much pain. *Br. J. Hosp. Med.*, January, pp. 63–6.

Miller, H. (1961) Accident neurosis. *Br. Med. J.*, **i**, 919–25; 992–8.

Murphy, M. (1989) Somatisation: embodying the problem. *Br. Med. J.*, **298**, 1331–2.

Pilowsky, I. (1969) Abnormal illness behaviour. *Br. J. Med. Psychol.*, **42**, 347–51.

Pilowsky, I. (1978) A general classification of abnormal illness behaviours. *Br. J. Med. Psychol.*, **51**, 131–7.

Pilowsky, I. (1985) Malingerophobia. *Med. J. Aust.*, **143**, 571–2.

Poore, G.V. (1878) Analysis of 75 cases of writer's cramp and impaired writing powers. *Trans. R. Med. Chirurg. Soc.*, **61**, 111–45.

Popper, K. (1959) *The Logic of Scientific Discovery*, 10th edn. Hutchinson, London. Popper, K. (1972) *Conjectures and Refutations*, 4th edn. Routledge and Kegan, London, pp. 228–9.

Quintner, J.L. and Cohen, M.L. (1994) Referred pain of peripheral nerve origin: an alternative to the 'myofascial pain' construct. *Clin. J. Pain*, **10**, 243–51.

Schofferman, J., Anderson, D., Hines, R. *et al.* (1992) Childhood psychological trauma correlates with unsuccessful lumbar spine surgery. *Spine*, **17**, S138–44.

Shacklock, M. (1995) Neurodynamics. *Physiotherapy*, **81**(1), 9–16.

Smythe, H.A. (1994) The C6–7 syndrome – clinical features and treatment response. *J. Rheumatol.*, **21**(8), 1520–6.

Travell, J.G. and Simons, D.G. (1983) Myofascial pain and dysfunction. In: *The Trigger Point Manual*. Williams & Wilkins, Baltimore, Md.

Tyrer, S.P. (1986) Learned pain behaviour. *Br. Med. J.*, **292**, 1–2.

Viikari-Juntura, E. (1984) Tenosynovitis, peritendinitis and the tennis elbow syndrome. *Scand. J. Work Environ. Health*, **10**, 443–9.

Waddell, G., Bircher, M., Finlayson, D. and Main, C.H. (1984) Symptoms and signs; physical disease or illness behaviour. *Br. Med. J.*, **289**, 739–41.

Waddell, G. (1987) A new clinical model for the treatment of low-back pain. Spine, **12**(7), 632–43.

Wall, P.D. (1994) Introduction to the edition after this one. In: *Textbook of Pain* (eds P.D. Wall and R. Melzack), 3rd edn. Churchill Livingstone, Edinburgh, pp. 1–7.

Williams, A.C. de C., Nicholas, M.K., Richardson, P.H., Pither, C.E. *et al.* (1993) Evaluation of a cognitive behavioural programme for rehabilitating patients with chronic pain. *Br. J. Gen. Pract.*, **43**, 513–18.

Williams, J.I. (1989) Illness behaviour to wellness behaviour. The 'School for Bravery' approach. *Physiotherapy*, **75**(1), 2–7.

Wolfe, F., Simons, D.G., Fricton, J. *et al.* (1992) The fibromyalgia and myofascial pain syndromes: a preliminary study of tender points and trigger points in patients with fibromyalgia, myofascial pain syndrome and no disease. *J. Rheumatol.*, **19**, 944–51.

3

Referred pain

The contemporary custom of assigning the cause of pain either to peripheral pathology or to mental pathology is too simple because it ignores the subtle dynamic properties of peripheral tissue and of the nervous system.

Patrick Wall (1994)

The main thrust of this chapter is an attempt to elucidate the pathogenesis of referred pain, thereby to offer a credible explanation for those clinical conditions, both spinal and peripheral, that give rise to upper limb pain and associated symptoms such as dysaesthesia. A far too simplistic view has often prevailed in the past: in particular, the combination of limb pain and axial spinal pain has been considered either to be radicular – the result of nerve root entrapment caused by an intervertebral disc prolapse or by degenerative stenosis of the intervertebral foramen, a potential surgical problem – or *referred* (inferring 'non-organicity', defying conventional understanding of nerve physiology, and not amenable to surgery).

A more thoughtful view of referred pain not only accords with information derived from a vast amount of research into nerve physiology and pathophysiology over the past decade and a half, but also with clinical experience. Somatic referred pain may be considered to be pain perceived in a region topographically distinct from the location of its nociceptive source. In strict neurological terms referred symptoms are perceived in a region innervated by peripheral nerves different from those that innervate the actual source of pain (Bogduk, 1992). An awareness of a wide spectrum of potential nociceptive sources of upper limb pain should stimulate a comprehensive clinical search for their presence. An appropriate management strategy may then be predicated upon a definitive clinical diagnosis.

Pain perception from lesions affecting the spine is usually mediated via the sinuvertebral (recurrent meningeal) nerves and/or the articular branches of the medial branches of the dorsal rami (Figure 3.1; see also Figure 6.4). The sinuvertebral nerves supply the posterior aspects of the intervertebral discs, the dura mater and the contents of the epidural space. Both the sinuvertebral nerves and the apophyseal articular nerves interconnect with corresponding nerves at adjacent segmental levels. Of particular relevance is the finding by Bogduk (1988) of the sensory innervation of the outer third of the annulus and adjacent tissues in the cervical spinal canal by the sinuvertebral nerve.

In the cervical spine, a contribution to the innervation of the intervertebral discs is made by the vertebral nerve which is derived predominantly from the sympathetic nervous system. The autonomic nervous system is also stimulated by the neurophysiological disturbances associated with spinal segmental dysfunction via the connections between the sympathetic chain and the dorsal root ganglia.

Peripheral nociceptive sources of arm pain are located in both the musculoskeletal system and the neurological system. The afferent nociceptive stimulus that initiates neural events giving rise to the common clinical findings of muscle hypertonus and areas of hyperalgesia may lie deeply in the soft tissues, such as the joint capsules, muscles and tendons or in the peripheral nerves. Of some considerable relevance to the differential diagnosis is the potential for peripheral neural symptoms to radiate proximally as well as distally.

In the following account the potential nociceptive sites involved in the perception of pain and associated symptoms in the neck, upper back and arm are identified.

Musculoskeletal origins

Bone

Whilst the classification of major spinal trauma is not relevant to this text, it should be noted that some spinal fractures give rise to symptoms in the upper back and in the upper limbs. Pathological fractures, for instance vertebral collapse in an osteoporotic spine (Figure 3.2), are often unrecognized by the unsuspecting clinician, but they may provide the initial stimulus to the development of neuropathic pain.

A *compression fracture* of a vertebral body is a not uncommon result of severe axial loading. The transitional region of the thoracolumbar junction is often affected – I can testify to a short-lived bout of back pain, caused by an L1 compression fracture, following a (feet first) collision with an Alpine ice wall when failing to control a downhill piste descent by toboggan. More frequently, spinal compression fractures result from jumping or falling from a height (a hazard in the construction industries) when they may be associated with lower limb trauma, such as ankle fractures.

A fall on to the upper back may result in a fracture of a proximal thoracic vertebra. Disturbed function of the intervertebral joints, the costovertebral joints and the anterior (sternocostal) joints of the thoracic cage (either as a consequence of a spinal compression fracture or as a result of a whiplash injury to the cervicodorsal spine) may give rise to pain that is referred to the arms as well as around the chest. Pain is often provoked by attempted abduction of the arms above shoulder height. An increased susceptibility to one of the work-related upper limb disorders may arise as a consequence of the adaptive postural responses to painful neck and upper back conditions.

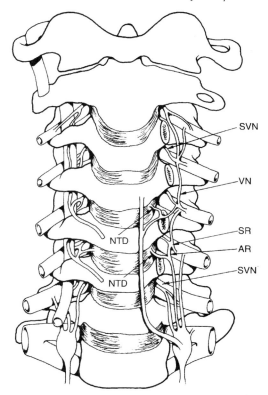

Figure 3.1 Anterior view of the cervical spine, demonstrating the origins of the C3 to C7 sinuvertebral nerves (SVN) from a somatic root (SR) and an autonomic root (AR). Also shown are nerves (NTD) to the C4–5 and C5–6 discs from the vertebral nerve (VN). (After Bogduk, 1988)

Referred pain patterns were identified by Kellgren (1939) and Inman and Saunders (1944) following noxious stimulation of *periosteum*. In these studies, periosteum was just one of several deep somatic structures that were investigated. (A further description is given below, see Muscles).

Posterior annulus fibrosus

Bogduk (1988) established that the cervical sinuvertebral nerves, together with branches of the vertebral nerve, supply the cervical intervertebral discs. Histological studies demonstrated the presence of nerve fibres as deeply as the outer third of the annulus fibrosus. He considered that this was sufficient evidence for the concept of primary disc pain.

Taylor and Kakulas (1993) have drawn attention to the prevalence of discogenic injury, including clefts in the anterior annulus adjacent to the anterior vertebral rim and traumatic lesions affecting the posterior margin of the annulus fibrosus (with localized annulus rupture), as a cause of significant, and commonly prolonged, neck pain after whiplash trauma to the cervical spine (Figure 3.3). They postulated that injured parts of the disc which normally have no innervation may acquire it by vascular and neural ingrowth into disc clefts. Under these circumstances, neck pain that radiates to the scapular region and to the shoulder may be due to primary disc/vertebral rim disturbances.

Unfortunately, the sensitivity of non-invasive investigative techniques such as magnetic resonance imaging in annular tears is modest at best: the presence of increased signal representing an annular tear is unreliable. Accordingly, the true incidence of significant pathological disruption of the annulus is unknown. Whiplash injuries, particularly acceleration injuries from rear-end vehicular collisions, may occur in the industrial setting (for instance with the use of fork-lift trucks or electric trolleys) and cause prolonged neck pain.

There is a further relevance to work in as much as the prognosis for whiplash injuries to the soft tissue supporting structures of the neck and upper back from whatever cause may be substantially affected by adverse spinal posture that is often associated with work that imposes further postural stresses upon these areas, such as prolonged use of a keyboard. Upon a background of discomfort and hyperalgesia in the shawl area (symptoms which, to a variable degree, are virtually endemic in keyboard workers), the additional stress following whiplash may precipitate more extensive, severe and prolonged upper limb pain.

Internal disc disruption

The concept of internal disc disruption (IDD) has developed over recent years and offers an organic explanation for low back pain and referred pain in the lower limb(s), and possibly for neck and upper limb pain, when there are no features of disc prolapse or facet joint disturbance. It is characterized by degradation of the nuclear matrix with the development of radial fissures, but with an intact annulus. The affected disc becomes painful as a result of chemical and/or mechanical irritation of the nerve endings in the outer annulus fibrosus (Bogduk, 1992). This situation is magnified if there is an annular tear, when leakage of nucleus pulposus material occurs into the annulus fibrosus.

Provocation discography has been adopted as the test for discogenic pain. It has been used widely in the lumbar spine, but it may have a useful role in the cervical spine too (Figure 3.4). Discography provokes pain in an abnormal disc, and post-discography CT may be used to reveal the typical disturbances of the disc architecture.

Longitudinal studies are required to evaluate the possible association between refractory spinal pain and disc degeneration as demonstrated by magnetic resonance imaging and, in particular, the relevance of internal disc

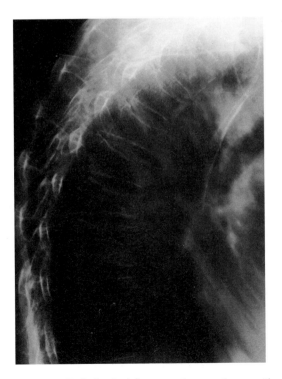

Figure 3.2 Pathological fractures in an osteoporotic spine may be unrecognized by the unsuspecting clinician

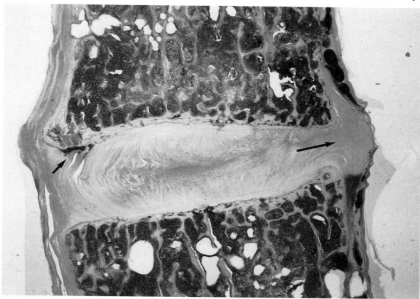

Figure 3.3 Annular disruptions may cause significant neck pain after whiplash trauma to the cervical spine. This sagittal section of a C6–7 disc from a 32-year-old man who died after a car accident reveals a small transverse cleft containing blood (short arrow) at the attachment of the anterior annulus to the vertebral rim, and a disc prolapse (long arrow) through the posterior annulus. (Courtesy of J.R. Taylor and B.A. Kakulas, Department of Neuropathology, Royal Perth Hospital)

disruption to painful conditions affecting the cervical spine. The possibility that internal chemical or mechanical changes within the intervertebral disc act as a primary noxious event in the development of the patho-neurophysiological phenomena that are postulated to be at the heart of both segmental (somatic) dysfunction and neuropathic arm pain is speculative, but attractive nevertheless.

Dura matter

The sinuvertebral nerves are known to innervate the cervical dura mater (Edgar, 1966; Bogduk and Marsland, 1988). The proximity of the dura to the posterior longitudinal ligament puts it at risk of compression from a posterior ('central') disc prolapse. Confirmatory evidence of indentation of the dura by this means comes from magnetic resonance imaging (Figure 3.5; see also Figure 3.6a).

In clinical practice, it has been accepted for several decades, particularly after the identification by Cyriax (1945) of the mechanism of dural pain in lumbago, that the dura mater is a sensitive structure which may be anaesthetized by epidural injections. For instance, symptomatic relief from back pain and/or sciatica that is secondary to a prolapse of the nucleus pulposus may be achieved by lumbar or caudal epidural injections of local anaesthetic and/or steroids. Cervical epidural injections too may be effective in refractory neck or arm pain.

From the cervical spine, radicular symptoms in a dermatomal segmental pattern in the upper limb are caused by compression of the dural investment of the emerging nerve root by disc herniation (Figure 3.6a) or (in the older patient) by intervertebral root canal stenosis (Figure 3.6b) (see below, Radicular pain).

Cyriax (1954) considered that 'extrasegmental' (non-segmental) reference was the result of dural pressure, either from a central or a lateral disc protrusion.

This mechanism explained the scapular pain so commonly experienced prior to the onset of a fully developed root palsy (and the associated segmental symptoms and signs).

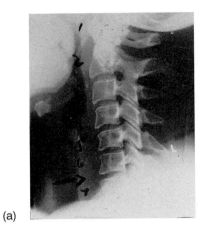

(a)

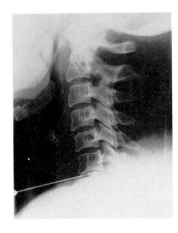

(b)

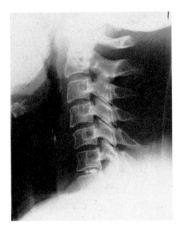

(c)

Figure 3.4 Provocation discography has been adopted as the test for discogenic pain. C6–7 discography is illustrated. (Courtesy of B.J. Preston, Department of Radiology, University Hospital, Nottingham)

Apophyseal (facet) joint

The work of Mooney and Robertson (1976) and of McCall *et al.* (1979) established the validity of what had been referred to as the 'facet joint syndrome' in the lumbar spine by Ghormley in 1933. Mooney and Robertson reinforced the concept of referred pain from the lumbar apophyseal joints, using facet joint arthrography, intra-articular injections of hypertonic saline, and pain pattern drawings in normal and abnormal subjects (Figure 3.7). Symptoms were relieved by intra-articular injections of local anaesthetic.

McCall reported on induced pain referral patterns from posterior lumbar segments in normal subjects, and followed this (Fairbank *et al.*, 1981) by using intra-articular apophyseal injections of local anaesthetic as a diagnostic aid in 'primary low-back pain syndromes'.

In an attempt to analyse the anatomical pain pathways in various pain syndromes in the neck and shoulder region, Bogduk (1982) provided a detailed description of the anatomy of the cervical dorsal rami and the innervation of the cervical apophyseal joints. The medial branches of the C4–8 dorsal rami supply the adjacent two apophyseal joints. Communication loops may link adjacent branches. The C3 dorsal ramus provides an articular branch to the C2–3 apophyseal joint, and an articular branch to the C3–4 joint via its deep

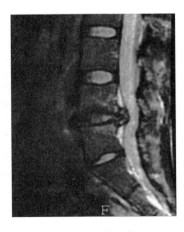

Figure 3.5 Dural compression from a central disc prolapse is demonstrated on this T2 weighted MRI scan of the lumbar spine. The high signal of the epidural fat is seen anterior to the thecal sac

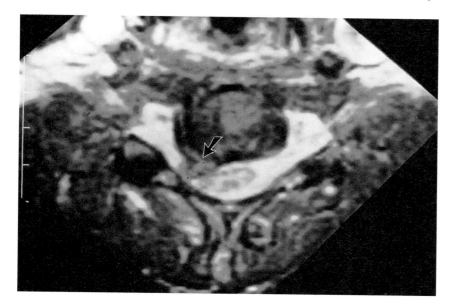

(a)

(b)

Figure 3.6 (*a*) MRI may reveal entrapment of the emerging nerve root. This T2 weighted axial image of C5–6 demonstrates a paracentral disc protrusion (*arrowed*) with impingement upon the nerve root and the spinal cord. (Courtesy of K. Bush) (*b*) Foraminal osteophytic hypertrophy may cause nerve root compression. (From M.A. Hutson, *Back Pain: Recognition and Management*. Butterworth–Heinemann, Oxford, 1993)

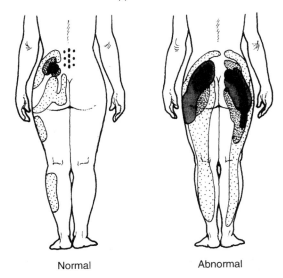

Normal   Abnormal

Figure 3.7 Pain referral patterns from stimulation of the lumbar facet joints in normal (asymptomatic) and abnormal (symptomatic) subjects. (After Mooney and Robertson, 1976)

medial branch. The atlanto-occipital joints are innervated by the C1 and C2 ventral rami.

More recently, Bogduk (1988) tested the hypothesis that the cervical apophyseal joints might be a significant source of pain in the neck and in the shawl area. Relief of symptoms was achieved in a significant number of patients with neck pain following cervical medial branch blocks and apophyseal joint blocks, revealing that the target joint was symptomatic (although not excluding the possibility of primary disc disease). In a further study, Bogduk and co-workers (Dwyer *et al.*, 1990) mapped out characteristic pain patterns following stimulation of apophyseal joints with contrast medium (Figure 3.8).

The facet joints are subject to osteoarthritis in the middle-aged and elderly. Degenerative changes in the facet joints, as elsewhere, cause reduced tolerance of physical activities that load the joints, but otherwise may give rise to spinal stiffness rather than pain. (Indeed, there is a poor correlation between degenerative changes on X-ray and the incidence of painful spinal syndromes.) However, it is logical to postulate that a painful synovial reaction may occur in a degenerate apophyseal joint, as in peripheral joints, as a response to work stresses and refer symptoms proximally (for example to the occiput) or distally.

The most likely cause of pain arising from disturbances of the facet joint in younger patients is somatic dysfunction (see below). In proximal cervical spinal joint dysfunction, symptoms are frequently referred to the suboccipital, occipital and facial areas. Occipital headaches are particularly common. Additionally, vertigo, diplopia, tinnitus, facial pains and temporomandibular joint dysfunction may arise. The Barré–Lieou syndrome (Barré, 1926) encompasses these and other symptoms that are possibly the result of stimulation of adjacent cranial nerve nuclei in the brain stem or stimulation of the autonomic system secondary to dysfunction at the craniocervical junction or the adjacent proximal cervical segments.

Following a whiplash injury to the neck discomfort from the soft tissue supporting structures of the mid/distal cervical spine, probably centred upon the apophyseal joints, is very commonly felt in the region of the scapular attachment of the proximal scapular fixator muscles at the superior vertebral angle of the scapula. It is often associated with a particularly pronounced myofascial trigger point – an example of secondary hyperalgesia (see below, Neuropathic pain). Referred pain, paraesthesia in a non-specific pattern and other symptoms that reflect sudomotor and vasomotor changes may be experienced in the arm, as far as the hand.

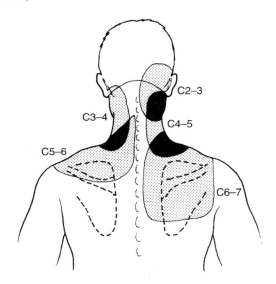

Figure 3.8 Pain patterns from cervical apophyseal joints. (After Dwyer *et al.*, 1990)

Similar symptoms in the neck and upper limb are not uncommonly experienced by assembly/production line factory workers and by keyboard operators. Intensive keyboard work that is unsupported by sound ergonomics is a particularly adverse prognostic factor following whiplash trauma: neck, shoulder and arm symptoms often persist for well over 12 months in clerical workers and typists.

The osteopathic interpretation of the observed axial and peripheral phenomena is that the features result from **somatic (reversible spinal joint) dysfunction**, the pathophysiology of which incorporates a 'facilitated cord segment' (indicating reflex pathoneurophysiological mechanisms). Somatic dysfunction is a functional segmental disturbance at the articulations between adjacent vertebrae. It is described as having two components – *localized segmental irritation* (accounting for localized muscle hypertonus, joint hypomobility and associated sensory features), and *peripheral segmental irritation* (which accounts for the referred symptoms in the limb). From my own observations I have also been aware of the frequent contribution to symptoms in the upper back and arms made by somatic dysfunction in the upper thoracic spine as well as the cervical spine.

The hypothesis of a neurophysiological cause for somatic dysfunction is strengthened by recent research from which has emerged the physiological concept of neural plasticity, and peripheral and central sensitization of the nervous system (see below, Neuropathic pain).

Cohen *et al.* (1992) propose that 'refractory cervicobrachial pain [type 2 WRULD in this text] is a *reflex neuropathic state* consequent upon *continuing afferent barrage* from nociceptors and mechanoreceptors in *anatomically relevant sites*' (my italics). Clearly, the intervertebral articulations and associated nerve roots may play a particularly important role in the perpetuation, and possibly in the development, of this disorder.

Muscles

Experimental evidence
For an understanding of the nature of referred pain from somatic origins it is illuminating to review the work of Kellgren and others who mapped the distribution of symptoms following stimulation of the deep somatic structures, including the paravertebral soft tissues, and a variety of limb and trunk muscles.

Kellgren (1938, 1939) systematically injected 6% hypertonic saline into the interspinous ligaments and paravertebral muscles below C4 in three subjects and noted the widespread but segmental distribution of referred pain and deep tenderness. Similar experiments were conducted following the injection of many different muscles of the trunk and limbs, including the scapular muscles and the muscles of the upper limb (Figure 3.9). Feinstein *et al.* (1954) expanded upon these observations and reproduced his findings following noxious stimulation of the axial (intervertebral and paravertebral) soft tissues from the atlanto-occipital area to the sacrum and also of peripheral muscles in both the upper and lower limbs. Pain patterns of a well-defined form emerged (Figure 3.10).

Other observations by Feinstein included the presence of hypoaesthesia ('hypoalgesia') adjacent to the midline and distributed irregularly throughout a segment, deep tenderness and muscle spasm, and autonomic symptoms (particularly after thoracic injections). Noxious stimulation of C6/7 evoked referred pain to the upper limb despite previous regional (brachial plexus) block or sympathetic denervation. Feinstein concluded that a central neural mechanism rather than peripheral nerve function was necessary for the expression of referred pain.

Bogduk (1988) also noted an area of hypoaesthesia with a surrounding hyperaesthetic border following local anaesthetic blocks of the medial branches of the dorsal rami in the cervical spine. Other researchers have confirmed that referred pain from injured tissue appears to depend on neural mechanisms as local anaesthesia blocks its expression. In the past the (subjective and 'semi-objective') findings of hypoaesthesia, deep muscle tenderness and autonomic symptoms have been recognized, if ill-understood, phenomena. However, the modern concept of neural pathophysiology offers a credible explanation for these common clinical features.

The term 'sclerotome' was introduced by Inman and Saunders (1944) to describe the segmental localization of symptoms in the

(a)   (b)

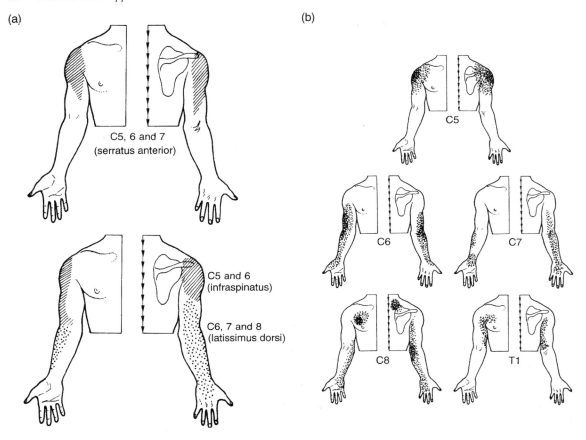

Figure 3.9 Kellgren (1938, 1939) noted the segmental distribution of referred pain and deep tenderness following injection of hypertonic saline into (*a*) muscles of the upper extremity and shoulder girdle, and (*b*) the interspinous ligaments. In (*b*) referred pain patterns are demonstrated for three subjects: vertical hatching, horizontal hatching and stippling

upper and lower limbs following noxious stimulation of periosteum, ligaments, joint capsules, tendons, fascia and muscles. They used the term to distinguish the pattern (and the overall concept) of referred pain from the 'dermatome' of nerve root stimulation. Both sclerotomes and dermatomes have segmental characteristics, but sclerotomes are more diffuse and are not associated with the specific sensory and motor disturbance of dermatomes. Sclerotomes do, however, have other associated features (such as sweating, pallor and nausea) that are probably the result of autonomic stimulation. Conceptually, the sclerotome is probably identical to the zone of peripheral segmental irritation, already

referred to in this text as a component of somatic dysfunction.

Interestingly, in their paper entitled 'Referred pain from skeletal structures' in 1944, Inman and Saunders noted the therapeutic value sometimes derived from injection of local anaesthetic 'at the trigger point which, by breaking the reflex arc, alleviates the pain'.

Muscle spasm/strain
Paraspinal muscle spasm may be observed clinically as a consequence of an intervertebral disc prolapse. It is protective in function and not under the conscious control of the patient. It is fallacious to consider that the muscle

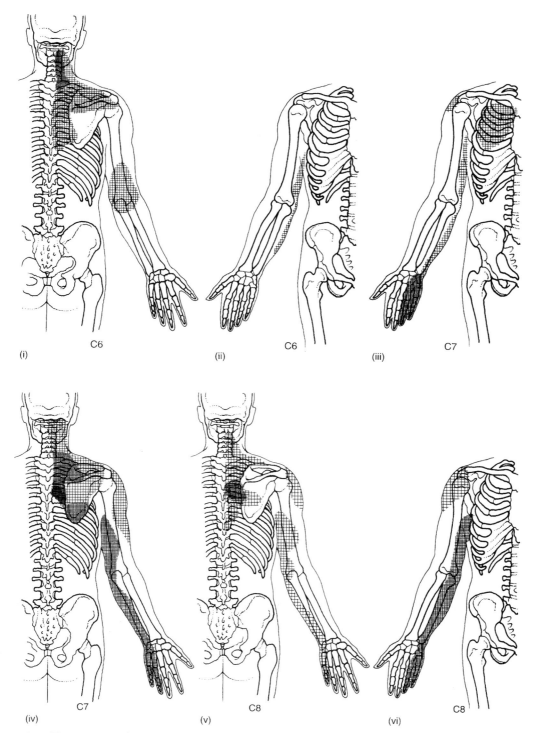

Figure 3.10 Feinstein *et al.* (1954) produced patterns of referred pain after intervertebral injections of hypertonic saline: C6–8 are demonstrated. At each level the areas of deep pain found in five subjects were superimposed

spasm is the sole or even a major contributor to the patient's pain.

A muscle 'strain' is a commonly encountered diagnosis. It suggests a tear at the musculotendinous junction (the most likely site for intrinsic muscle injury) or at its bony attachment, both of which are found in peripheral muscle injuries. However, it is most unlikely that a diagnosis of 'muscle strain' affecting the paraspinal muscles is the correct diagnosis in cases of neckache or low backache, acute or chronic, other than perhaps in a very small percentage of patients.

It is much more likely that in refractory neck and arm pain the primary nociceptive stimulus arises in the articular and periarticular structures of the spine (the facet joints and their associated ligaments) or in the nerve roots or their sheaths. Under these circumstances, as a consequence of spinal joint dysfunction, the tenderness identified in the muscles in the paraspinal region, around the pectoral girdle and in the arm is due to *secondary hyperalgesia*.

Myofascial pain

The concept of myofascial pain in which tender **trigger points** (TPs or TrPs) are a primary feature has been proposed and elaborated upon by Travell and Simons (1983). A regional myofascial pain syndrome (MPS) incorporates this concept and defines a trigger point as '*a hyperirritable spot, usually within a taut band of skeletal muscle or in the muscle's fascia, that is painful on compression and that can give rise to characteristic referred pain, tenderness, and autonomic phenomena*'. The authors differentiate trigger points from tender points (which are generally accepted to be a widespread feature of fibromyalgia) by conferring on trigger points exclusively the palpable taut bands with local twitch responses. Additionally, trigger points are considered to be more likely to produce referred pain on palpation.

It is apparent that a referred pain pattern is an essential component of the MPS concept. A characteristic reference zone of deep aching pain is located some distance from the trigger point. Confirmation (to both patient and examiner) that the trigger point is the source of pain is reproduction of the patient's pain pattern by pressure on the trigger point. *The Trigger Point Manual* (Travell and Simons, 1983) is a veritable encyclopaedia of referred pain patterns from single-muscle myofascial

pain syndromes. Of particular relevance to the upper limb (Figure 3.11) are:

(a) the pain patterns from trigger points in the neck and pectoral girdle muscles, including:
  • the **scaleni** (affecting the radial aspect of the arm as far as the radial three digits);
  • the **supraspinatus** (affecting the lateral aspect of the elbow and adjacent forearm, in addition to the shoulder);
  • the **infraspinatus** (affecting the upper arm predominantly but including the radial aspect of the arm and hand);
(b) the pain patterns from trigger points in the arm muscles, including:
  • the **supinator** (affecting the web between the first and second digits in addition to the lateral elbow);
  • the **extensores carpi radialis** (affecting the dorsum of the wrist and hand in addition to the lateral elbow);
  • the **first dorsal interosseous** (affecting the radial aspect of the index finger particularly).

In contrast to the myofascial pain concept, an equally attractive pathophysiological hypothesis for tender muscle is that of secondary hyperalgesia (described further in the section on 'Neuropathic pain' later in the chapter). When trigger points are relatively isolated (topographically) on clinical examination they are often associated with spinal conditions, either a disc prolapse giving rise to dural irritation or somatic (reversible spinal joint) dysfunction. *Such trigger points (or hyperalgesic zones) are found commonly in the proximal scapular fixator muscles (trapezius and levator scapulae) when they are secondary to cervical and cervicodorsal junctional spinal conditions.* When found in the glutei, piriformis and psoas muscles they are secondary to lumbar or sacroiliac conditions.

Disseminated foci of muscle hypertonus or 'tender points' (probably representing areas of secondary hyperalgesia) are a marked feature of type 2 (the diffuse form) WRULD. Generalized tender points, occurring in many muscle groups bilaterally and affecting the lower half of the body as well as the upper limbs, are a feature of fibromyalgia.

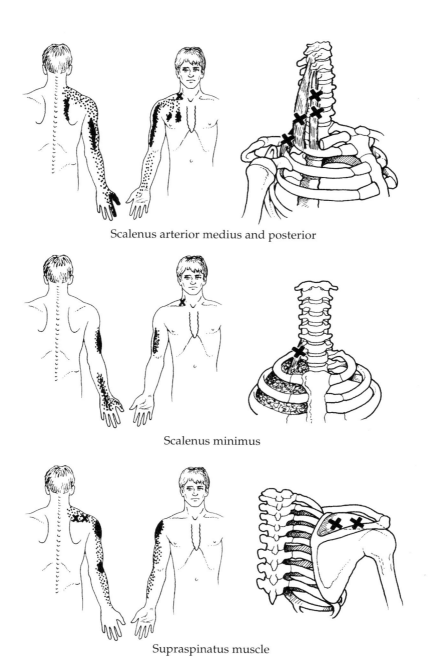

Scalenus arterior medius and posterior

Scalenus minimus

Supraspinatus muscle

Figure 3.11 Location of trigger points and referred pain patterns from some of the neck, shoulder girdle and arm muscles: scaleni, supraspinatus, infraspinatus, supinator, extensores carpi radialis and first dorsal interosseous. (After Travell and Simons, 1983) (continued overleaf)

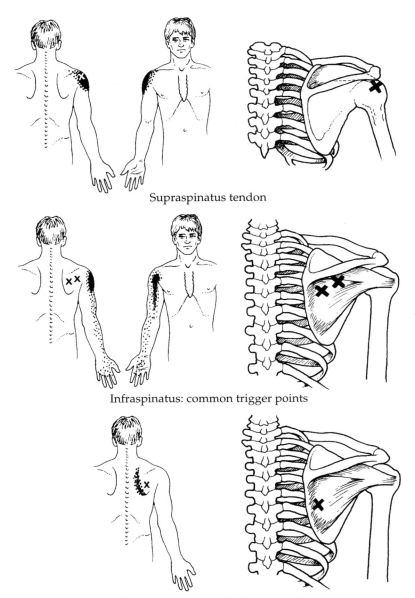

Supraspinatus tendon

Infraspinatus: common trigger points

Infraspinatus: unusual trigger points

Figure 3.11 (continued)

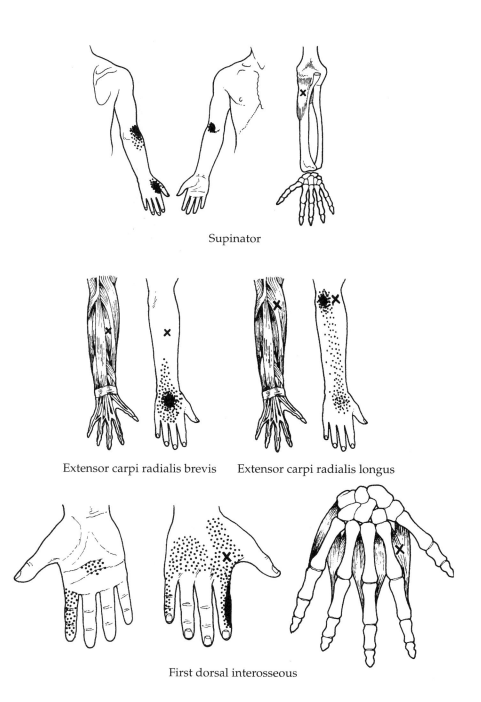

Supinator

Extensor carpi radialis brevis   Extensor carpi radialis longus

First dorsal interosseous

Figure 3.11 (continued)

Of the two described hypotheses for tender muscle – the myofascial pain syndrome and secondary hyperalgesia – experimental studies favour the latter. However, the pathophysiology of trigger points remains conjectural. Muscle biopsy studies of trigger points by light microscopy, histochemistry or electron microscopy have not demonstrated consistent abnormalities. Needle electromyography (EMG) has also produced variable results, but in a study by Hubbard and Berkoff (1993) sustained spontaneous (EMG) activity was found in a 1–2 mm nidus of all trigger points in the upper trapezius (but was not present in non-trigger points) in patients with headache, neck and shoulder pain. The authors hypothesized that 'trigger points are caused by sympathetically activated intrafusal contraction . . . giving rise to involuntary low-grade but symptomatic muscle tension'. Sympathetic activity was deemed 'to explain the autonomic symptoms associated with trigger points and to provide a mechanism by which local injury and nociception causes local tension, and by which emotional factors cause widespread tension and pain'.

Muscle overuse

Hunter Fry, from a background of considerable experience of musicians' injuries in Australia, considers that injurious change can be brought about in muscle by prolonged submaximal contraction. He considers that 'overuse syndrome' in musicians and keyboard operators for instance is 'a condition of pain and loss of function of muscles and ligaments which have been subjected to excessive or unaccustomed use' (Fry, 1986).

He supports his hypothesis by histopathological evidence of significant changes in the first dorsal interosseous muscles of keyboard operators; such changes included loss of type 2 fibres, type 1 fibre grouping, significant fibre hypertrophy, mitochondrial lesions and a number of other ultramicroscopic findings (Dennett and Fry, 1988). Unfortunately, these findings have not been repeated. By contrast, the morphological changes such as Z-disc disruption and infiltration of mononuclear cells in muscles sampled after unaccustomed and frequent eccentric contractions (in a number of studies) are in patients who make an early recovery from acute 'injury', *and do not suffer from chronic pain*.

Prolonged submaximal muscle contraction is also considered to be the basis of overuse injury, as observed in the early stages of the diffuse form of WRULD, by the Occupational Safety and Health Service in New Zealand. It has been postulated that sustained muscle contraction generates a nociceptive stimulus as a result of a compromised microcirculation and oxygen lack (Wigley *et al.*, 1992). Waste products such as lactic acid and pyruvic acid accumulate. Additionally, chemicals such as prostaglandins and bradykinin and other possible neurotransmitters are produced, leading to neural sensitization. Pain is accompanied by further muscle tension/spasm, and a self-sustaining cycle of muscle tension is produced. The advocates of this hypothesis concede that widespread referral of pain indicates the onset of a chronic pain syndrome (as described later).

From my own experience in the field of sports injuries (Hutson, 1996) and musculoskeletal conditions in general, I am unable to support the concept of overuse injury to contractile structures to account for such diffuse and diverse symptoms and signs as are found in the diffuse form of WRULD. Most sporting activities are dependent upon repetitive eccentric muscle contractions – a far cry from the sustained isometric contractions associated with constrained postures in many occupations. Undoubtedly, the concept of sustained muscle tension as a potential *primary nociceptive stimulus* in the earliest stages of type 2 WRULD cannot be dismissed without serious consideration.

Tendons

Tendinopathies are discussed in Chapter 5. Although the role of tendinitis in the early stages of type 2 WRULD is conjectural, anecdotal evidence suggests that many patients recall a sudden 'pull', 'twang', or 'tear' in the hand, wrist or forearm as the earliest symptom prior to a more gradual intensification and dissemination of discomfort. It is not unusual for these early symptoms to be accompanied by tingling and numbness distally, suggesting that an inflammatory response associated with a relatively minor tendon injury provokes neural irritation.

An analogy with overuse injury in sport is useful once more. Repetitive musculotendinous activity involving the upper limb in a sportsman may be compared with similar hand–arm activity in an industrial worker who is engaged in rapid, repetitive work. The delicate state of biological adaptation to physical stress may be compromised by a relatively small increase in load to a level that causes excessive microscopic tissue degradation and a low grade tendinitis. Primary afferent nociceptive stimulation from within the affected tendon results in pain which may be referred (proximally as well as distally) along the limb in the same fashion as referred pain from muscle.

Ligaments

Kellgren (1938, 1939) injected hypertonic saline into the interspinous ligaments of the cervical spine and observed pain patterns in the neck, shoulder girdle and arm. Hackett (1956) introduced noxious chemicals to the lumbosacral and sacroiliac ligaments and also observed reproducible pain patterns in the back, pelvis and leg. Back pain, local tenderness and referred pain may all be relieved by localized ligamentous injections of local anaesthetic (Steindler and Luck, 1938).

Clinically, the concept of chronic ligamentous strain of the supraspinous or interspinous ligaments in both sexes, and the sacroiliac ligaments in women, as a cause of low back and pseudoradicular pain is attractive. It is supported by the experience in clinical practice of prolonged relief of symptoms in some cases following interspinous injections of steroid and local anaesthetic.

It is logical to postulate that stimulation of primary afferent nociceptor nerve endings in the intervertebral ligaments situated in the cervical and proximal thoracic spines may make a contribution to the development of pathological pain in the upper limb.

Neural origins

Radicular pain

In the cervical spine the nerve root sheath is susceptible to traction (for instance by being stretched over a posterolateral disc herniation) and also to compression; in the latter circumstance any space-occupying tissue, for instance extruded disc material or bony encroachment into the intervertebral foramen, may 'nip' the nerve root, commonly during extension or ipsilateral side flexion of the cervical spine.

Established techniques to detect dural tension in the lower limb include the straight leg raise test, the femoral nerve stretch test and the slump test; they are positive when the relevant root sheath is tethered. With respect to the upper limb, Elvey (1986) has devised a brachial plexus tension test (BPTT) which is comparable as a neural tension test for the C5–7 nerve roots to the conventional aforementioned tests for the lumbar/sacral roots. Adverse neural tension has been inculpated in the pathogenesis of type 2 WRULD by Quintner and Elvey (1993) (see below, Neuropathic pain).

In the cervical spine the roots most commonly affected by entrapment are C6 and C7 (arising from C5/6 and C6/7 disc prolapses respectively), although lesions proximally and distally, affecting the C5 and C8 roots, are not uncommon. Occasionally, in the middle-aged as well as in old age, cord compression occurs at one or more segmental levels. Thickening of the ligamentum flavum and facet joint hypertrophy are the primary causes of this degenerative form of spinal stenosis. The signs of cord compression (detected by a neurological examination of the lower limbs) in addition to root entrapment should be sought on clinical examination: sometimes, symptoms from compression of the long tracts (such as difficulty walking and discomfort in the legs from muscle spasticity) may be the presenting features.

Radicular symptoms are ('classically') experienced along dermatomes which are reproduced in most textbooks of general medicine, orthopaedics and neurology. Disappointingly, however, many patients' capacity for spatial discrimination of peripheral symptoms, for instance when questioned about the distribution of their pain and paraesthesiae, is poor. Additionally, the sensory component of their radicular symptomatology may not be a prominent feature, thereby reducing the diagnostic value of this aspect of history-taking. When paraesthesiae and numbness are present, however, and particularly when motor signs are absent, their distribution may be the most sensitive guide to the affected level.

The presence of peripheral paraesthesiae and numbness in association with limb pain is often taken to be indicative of root entrapment (and therefore radicular in type). Although cutaneous sensory impairment may indeed be detected objectively in these circumstances, thereby confirming neural compression, similar symptoms could be pseudoradicular (that is, referred) in nature, particularly when combined with a 'burning' sensation (see below). Sensory phenomena may also result from compression/irritation of nerve trunks some distance from the spine (for instance, from brachial plexus trauma, or as a component of thoracic outlet syndrome), or from peripheral entrapment neuropathy.

True radicular pain is often severe and may be present nocturnally. Recumbency may not relieve the pain, as testified by the majority of patients with cervical nerve root entrapment who commonly suffer from disturbed nights until critical regression of the prolapsed disc material occurs. Symptoms are activity-dependent and posture-dependent, their longevity determined by the nature of the causative spinal pathology.

Peripheral neural pain

Peripheral nerve entrapment syndromes and their characteristic sensory (and motor) deficits are described in Chapter 5. Less 'classical' sensory disturbances in the hand and arm may be a manifestation of referred phenomena. A brief historical reflection is useful.

The preferential use of the terms 'neurosis', 'neuralgia', or 'neuritis' reflects the changing nosological attitudes to nerve-derived pain over the past century. Gowers (1892) championed the term 'occupational neurosis' to describe upper limb disorders associated with occupational factors. The designation 'neurosis' implied that there was no known organic lesion affecting the nervous system; instead, the concepts of central (nervous system) dysfunction and neurasthenia, the latter indicating a constitutional vulnerability to stressful life factors, were in vogue. Distinction was made between the spasmodic (motor) and neuralgic (sensory) forms of occupational neurosis.

In the early years of the twentieth century it became apparent that some types of occupational neurosis were a result of derangement of peripheral nerves. 'Neuritis' was coined, but subsequently rejected when it became apparent that no inflammatory condition existed. The term *'neuropathy'* is now used to describe a significant loss of function of a nerve or nerves, as in diabetic neuropathy or the Guillain–Barré syndrome, and *'nerve entrapment'* to denote those conditions in which there is considerable extrinsic (mechanical) pressure on a nerve.

The term 'neuralgia' was introduced to denote the presence of sensory symptoms such as burning, tingling, numbness and a feeling of coldness or swelling. Objective changes in cutaneous sensibility are often not present, or are only slight. 'Dysaesthesia' is perhaps the equivalent modern descriptor of these peripheral symptoms, though 'nerve trunk' pain which often has a deep aching quality may coexist with dysaesthesiae. The current hypothesis of a neurogenic cause for the diffuse variety of work-related arm pain (type 2 WRULD) has overtaken the previous concept of neuralgic pain (see below, Neuropathic pain).

Pathophysiological changes within the nervous system may occur both peripherally and centrally following peripheral nerve damage (Devor and Rappaport, 1990). Peripheral neural pain is probably perceived following activation of nociceptors within the connective tissue of a nerve (the nervi nervorum) at the site of nerve entrapment. Additionally, there may be activation of nociceptors or mechanoreceptors within the nerve sheath. Consequential sensorineural processing accounts for *physiological pain* of peripheral nerve origin. If peripheral sensitization occurs (see under Neuropathic pain) the neuralgic symptoms may be accompanied by hyperaesthesiae (allodynia and hyperalgesia).

The deep aching pain often associated with specific areas of tenderness, radiating *proximally* from a peripheral nerve entrapment, was recognized by Kopell and Thompson (1963). This constitutes a form of *referred pain of peripheral neural origin*. The proferred explanation, namely that secondary hyperalgesia in the muscles throughout the upper limb reflects the segmental relationship to the injured nerve, is probably simplistic.

The role of neural plasticity in nociceptive (referred) pain and dysaesthesiae

Referred phenomena

Peripheral tissue damage typically produces pain and (primary) hyperalgesia that is associated with increased sensitivity to noxious stimulation at the site of injury. Not uncommonly, damage to peripheral soft tissues or to nerves produces pain and secondary hyperalgesia that extends well beyond the site of injury – **referred** pain and tenderness. Peripheral neural mechanisms are inculpated in this process, which results in a number of characteristic features, collectively labelled dysaesthesiae:

- hyperaesthesia (sensory hypersensitivity, including allodynia and hyperalgesia);
- hypoaesthesia;
- autonomic nervous system changes.

'Allodynia' is the term given to the state of hypersensitivity (a lowered threshold) to non-noxious stimuli (including touch and gentle palpatory examination techniques) experienced by patients with heightened excitability of the nervous system. When widespread the term 'allopathia' is sometimes used. Frankly neuralgic symptoms (e.g. feelings of burning, electric shocks, pins and needles) may accompany such increased sensitivity to touch.

'Hyperalgesia' is defined as an abnormally pronounced response to noxious stimuli – an amplification of responsiveness – such as may be exhibited following firm digital pressure during palpatory examination techniques (mechanical hyperalgesia) or following thermal stimuli (thermal hyperalgesia).

The presence of primary hyperalgesia and allodynia in the zone immediately adjacent to the injury site is a response to tissue damage and should be considered protective in nature. When situated some distance from the site of injury such responses are often described as 'inappropriate'. However, such zones of secondary hyperalgesia are usually a manifestation of a sensitized central nervous system. In a minority of patients these hyperalgesic and allopathic features are accompanied by features of abnormal illness behaviour; these behavioural characteristics are also frequently labelled as 'inappropriate' (with respect to the precipitating stimulus), but in fact represent behavioural maladjustment rather than malingering.

Hypoaesthesia (a subjective feeling of numbness) may be detected as a well-localized zone close to the (axial) source of the nociceptive stimulation. The inexperienced practitioner may be bemused when unexpected symptoms of this type are volunteered by patients. Appraisal of the skin texture (for evidence of sudomotor changes) and the state of skin sensitivity (for hypoaesthesia or hyperaesthesia) should be an essential and routine part of any musculoskeletal examination.

In most textbooks of osteopathic medicine are to be found references to altered texture of the skin and subcutaneous tissues. Segmental sweating changes and subcutaneous oedema are probably responsible for the signs of 'skin drag' and abnormal 'skin rolling' that are common features of somatic (spinal) dysfunction. I recommend the routine use of skin rolling during a musculoskeletal examination. A localized area of abnormal tissue texture and hyperaesthesia is a common finding in lesions of the thoracic spine in particular, but is not specific to 'mechanical' dysfunctional states; it may also occur in association with spinal metastases, and when generalized it is a feature (in association with myofascial trigger or tender points) of fibromyalgia.

Pathoneurophysiology

A satisfactory hypothesis for the pathogenesis of upper limb pain referred from an identifiable focus in the neck or arm must explain the frequency of allodynia and hyperalgesia. Neural plasticity is the most credible hypothesis. It has been argued that referred pain from an injured region depends on the *misinterpretation* of nociceptive processing along axons which also branch to the uninjured area. Alternatively, referred pain may result from convergence of axons from injured and non-injured regions on dorsal horn cells.

However, central nervous system changes are suggested by the findings that referred pain and hyperalgesia spread to areas which do not share the same dermatome (Coderre *et al.*, 1993). The spatial extent of hypersensitivity is explored further in the next section.

Neuropathic pain

A neurogenic hypothesis must explain the clinical features of the disorder labelled type 2 WRULD in this text. These features include the diffuse spread of pain, the widespread allodynia and articular hyperalgesia, the tender (or 'trigger') points and hypertonus in muscle, the sensory and other neuralgic features, the motor weakness without wasting, the vasomotor symptoms and signs, the features of focal dystonia, and the *chronicity and refractoriness* of many cases. Type 2 WRULD is also frequently referred to as 'repetitive strain injury' or 'diffuse overuse syndrome' or 'refractory cervicobrachial pain syndrome' (by Cohen, Quintner and colleagues in Australia whose researches and opinions in recent years have done much to translate the concept of pathological pain developed by Clifford Woolf to the pathogenesis of occupational neck and arm pain).

Physiological pain

Under normal circumstances, physiological pain is the consequence of the activation of small diameter, thinly myelinated A delta and unmyelinated C nociceptive afferents with slow conduction velocities by high intensity noxious stimuli. Such stimuli include pinprick, firm pressure, pinch, excessive heat or cold, and abrasions to the skin. Neural processing occurs in the spinal cord, and involves both nociceptive specific neurones and others that are activated by low and high intensity stimuli (wide dynamic range neurones). This results in a direct relationship between the intensity of the stimulus – mechanical, thermal or chemical – and the subjective experience of pain.

Furthermore, other aspects of noxious stimuli such as location and duration are perceived accurately by the brain. The result is the typical flexion withdrawal response in unison with the sensation of pain and a general autonomic response. *Primary hyperalgesia* is localized to the zone immediately surrounding the injury site. Physiological pain is therefore considered to be nociceptor-mediated pain.

Pathological pain

The stimulus to the development of the concept of pathological (chronic) pain was the gate control theory of Melzack and Wall (1965). The focus of the modulation of pain pathways and the perception of pain became the dorsal horn neurones of the spinal cord. Modulation is affected by the relative amount of small and large fibre afferent input, by local systems and by descending neuronal pathways. Subsequently, Woolf (1983), working from his laboratory at University College, London, in the 1980s, described the concept of central sensitization: a feature of the plasticity of the central nervous system.

Following peripheral soft tissue or nerve injury, *sensory hypersensitivity* to both noxious and some non-noxious stimuli arises – a disruption of normal sensory neural processing mechanisms manifesting clinically as allodynia and hyperalgesia. An 'inflammatory soup' of chemicals causes an alteration in the transduction properties of primary high threshold afferent nociceptors in the vicinity of the injury, resulting in their activation by low intensity stimuli (**peripheral sensitization**) (Figure 3.12). Additionally, a subpopulation of afferents that are normally 'silent' begin to respond to mechanical or thermal stimuli. In its acute form this type of neurophysiological response to inflammation, characterized by a zone of primary hyperalgesia, promotes physiological repair processes and may be seen to have a useful and protective function.

Two aspects of post-traumatic pain hypersensitivity cannot be accounted for by a simple change in the transduction sensitivity of peripheral nociceptors. The first is the spatial extent of the hypersensitivity, and the second is the capacity of low threshold mechanoreceptors to produce pain (Woolf, 1991). The explanation for these observations is **central sensitization** (Figure 3.13). Alterations in the response properties of WDR (*wide dynamic range*) neurones in the dorsal horn are triggered by repetitive stimulation of small diameter primary afferent fibres. This results in an increase in their excitability (an abnormally high rate of firing) in response to large diameter, A beta low threshold myelinated afferents. Additionally, changes of activity in dorsal horn neurones known as *'wind–up'* occur, whereby sustained or repetitive inputs from nociceptive C fibres lead to a progressive

PERIPHERAL SENSITIZATION

(Nociceptor-mediated pain)

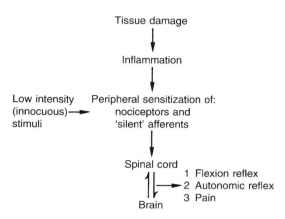

Figure 3.12 Diagrammatic representation of peripheral sensitization

increase in the discharge produced by further stimuli (Kidd *et al.*, 1996).

Under normal circumstances the activation of A beta afferents by tactile stimuli, pressure to deep tissue and movements of joints does not produce pain. Once wind–up and central hyperexcitability are established, however, there is an increase in response to standard stimuli, an expansion in the size of receptive fields and a reduction in threshold (Woolf, 1991).

Mechanical pain sensitivity may be viewed as the consequence of a misinterpretation of normal sensory inputs which are not part of the nociceptive system and which do not normally generate pain. If this situation persists for longer than three months (a somewhat arbitrary period, but one that is convenient for classification) the neuropathic pain then appears to lose any protective function and becomes truly abnormal.

Although the change of excitability of the dorsal horn cells is triggered by an afferent barrage (particularly the unmyelinated C afferents arising in deep tissue), it is maintained by central mechanisms. Following the release of peptides from the terminals of unmyelinated afferents, there are prolonged changes in the membrane and chemistry of the dorsal horn cells. The excitatory amino acids such as glutamate are involved in the activation of the N-methyl-D-aspartate (NMDA) receptor in the cells. Substance P acts

as a neuromodulator. Additionally, the prolonged changes may be maintained by 'a trickle of abnormal afferent inputs' (Wall, 1991). A third mechanism appears to be the chameleon-like nature of the dorsal horn cells: nociceptive specific cells undergo morphological change to become convergent (WDR) cells. Whatever the mechanisms of maintenance, once central sensitization has developed it persists for a relatively long time after the initiating cause has disappeared.

Application to neck and arm pain

It is postulated that type 2 WRULD is, in effect, a form of neuropathic arm pain (NAP) – a reflex neuropathic state characterized by prolonged excitation of WDR neurones in the dorsal horns consequent upon sustained afferent activity in nociceptors and mechanoreceptors in somatic structures (Cohen *et al.*, 1992). These anatomical sites probably include the spinal apophyseal joints, the muscles and joints in the upper limb, and the peripheral nerves and nerve roots. Constrained work postures and repetitive use of the hand and arm are commonly major contributors to the persistent afferent barrage. Chronicity may also be due to the *lack of supervening modulation* for the development of a cyclical disturbance in which hyperalgesic muscle maintains the sensitized state of the central nervous system at a segmental spinal level (Hancock, 1995).

CENTRAL SENSITIZATION

(A fibre-mediated pain)

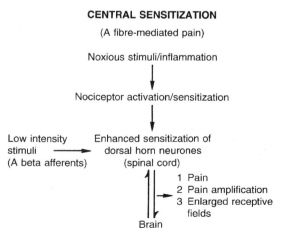

Figure 3.13 In central sensitization there is an increase in the excitability of wide dynamic range neurones in the dorsal horn in response to A beta low threshold afferents

By contrast, Quintner and Elvey (1993) postulate that mechanical tension upon neural structures, either distally (for instance at the wrist) or proximally (for instance within the cervical spine), generates abnormal discharges within the nervous system, and that such neural entrapment is the primary precipitating event in the development of chronic upper limb pain. Cohen and his co-workers and Quintner and Elvey have contributed significantly to the overall concept that chronic diffuse upper limb pain, on both clinical and neurophysiological grounds, is due to **secondary hyperalgesia**. Secondary hyperalgesia is observed some distance from the site of injury, in tissue that is innervated by peripheral nerves in the same or adjacent segments to that of the noxious stimulus.

This neuropathic state explains the 'conversion' of normally painless mechanoreceptor activity to a nociceptive state, the projection of paraesthesiae into extended receptive fields and the amplification of normal sensory input at the dorsal horn level giving rise to allodynia, hyperalgesia and hyperpathia (Cohen *et al.*, 1992). The concept of neuropathic arm pain offers a rational explanation for the referred phenomena described in this chapter, such as the association between muscle tenderness and dural irritation (as postulated by Cyriax); between peripheral zones of irritation and somatic dysfunction (a basic osteopathic concept); and between TPs and regional pain syndromes (such as type 2 WRULD).

In summary, although debate continues on whether primary somatic tissue damage or primary neural damage is a prerequisite to the development of neural sensitization, the diversity of the symptoms and signs strongly suggests that type 2 WRULD is a form of neuropathic arm pain (NAP) – caused by peripheral and central sensitization of the nervous system. Secondary motor, sensory and sympathetic responses are expressions of neural excitation.

References

Barré, J.A. (1926) Sur un syndrome sympathique cervical postérieure et sa cause fréquente: l'arthrite cervicale. *Rev. Neurol.*, **33**, 1246.

Bogduk, N. (1982) The clinical anatomy of the cervical dorsal rami. *Spine*, **7**, 319–30.

Bogduk, N. (1988) The innervation of the cervical intervertebral discs. *Spine*, **13**, 2–8.

Bogduk, N. (1992) The causes of low back pain. *Med. J. Aust.*, **156**, 151–3.

Bogduk, N. and Marsland, A. (1988) The cervical zygapophyseal joints as a source of neck pain. *Spine*, **13**, 610–17.

Coderre, T.J., Katz, J., Vaccarino, A.L. and Melzack, R. (1993) Contribution of central neuroplasticity to pathological pain: review of clinical and experimental evidence. *Pain*, **52**, 259–85.

Cohen, M.L., Arroyo, J.F., Champion, G.D. and Browne, C.D. (1992) In search of the pathogenesis of refractory cervicobrachial pain syndrome. *Med. J. Aust.*, **156**, 432–6.

Cyriax, J. (1945) Lumbago: mechanism of dural pain. *Lancet*, **ii**, 427–9.

Cyriax, J. (1954) *Textbook of Orthopaedic Medicine*. Cassell, London.

Dennett, X. and Fry, H.J.H. (1988) Overuse syndrome: a muscle biopsy study. *Lancet*, **i**, 905–8.

Devor, M. and Rappaport, Z.H. (1990) Pain and the pathophysiology of the damaged nerve. In *Pain Syndromes in Neurology* (ed. H.L. Fields), Butterworth–Heinemann, Oxford, pp. 47–83.

Dwyer, A., Aprill, C. and Bogduk, N. (1990) Cervical zygapophyseal joint pain patterns. *Spine*, **15**, 453–61.

Edgar, M.A. and Nundy, S. (1966) Innervation of the spinal dura mater. *J. Neurol. Neurosurg. Psychiat.*, **29**, 530–4.

Elvey, R.L. (1986) Treatment of arm pain associated with abnormal brachial plexus tension. *Aust. J. Physiother.*, **32**, 225–30.

Fairbank, J.C.T., Park, W.M., McCall, I.W. and O'Brien, J.P. (1981) Apophyseal joint injection of local anaesthetic as a diagnostic aid in primary low-back pain syndromes. *Spine*, **6**, 598–605.

Feinstein, B., Langton, J.N.K., Jameson, R.M. *et al.* (1954) Experiments on pain referred from deep somatic tissues. *J. Bone Joint Surg.*, **36A**, 981–97.

Fry, H.H. (1986) Overuse syndrome in musicians: prevention and management. *Lancet*, **ii**, 728–31.

Ghormley, R.K. (1933) Low back pain with special reference to the articular facets, with presentation of an operative procedure. *JAMA*, **101**, 1773–7.

Gowers, W.R. (1892) *A Manual of Diseases of the Nervous System*, 2nd edn. J. & A. Churchill, London, pp. 710–30.

Hackett, G.S., (1956) *Joint Ligament Relaxation Treated by Fibro-osseous Proliferation*. Charles C. Thomas, Springfield, Ill.

Hancock, J. (1995) Comments on Barnsley *et al.* [Barnsley *et al.* (1994) Clinical review: whiplash injury. *Pain*, **58**, 283–307]. *Pain*, **61**, 487–95.

Hubbard, D.R. and Berkoff, G.M. (1993) Myofascial trigger points show spontaneous needle EMG activity. *Spine*, **18**(13), 1803–7.

Hutson, M.A. (1996) *Sports Injuries: Recognition and Management*, 2nd edn. Oxford, Oxford University Press.

Inman, V.T. and Saunders, J.B. de C. (1944) Referred pain from skeletal structures. *J. Nerv. Ment. Dis.*, **99**, 660–7.

Kellgren, J.H. (1938) Observations on referred pain arising from muscle. *Clin.Sci.*, **3**, 175–90.

Kellgren, J.H. (1939) On the description of pain arising from deep somatic structures with charts of segmental pain areas. *Clin. Sci.*, **4**, 35–46.

Kidd, B.L., Morris, V.H. and Urban, L. (1996) Pathophysiology of joint pain. *Ann. Rheum. Dis.*, **55**, 276–83.

Kopell, H.P. and Thompson, W.A.L. (1963) *Peripheral Entrapment Neuropathies*. Williams and Wilkins, Baltimore.

McCall, I.W., Park, W.M., and O'Brien, J.P. (1979) Induced pain referral from posterior lumbar elements in normal subjects. *Spine*, **4**, 441–6.

Melzack, R. and Wall, P.D. (1965) Pain mechanisms: a new theory. *Science*, **150**, 971–8.

Mooney, V. and Robertson, J. (1976) The facet syndrome. *Clin. Orthop.*, **115**, 149–56.

Quintner, J.L. and Elvey, R.L. (1991) The neurogenic hypothesis of RSI. In: Bammer, G. (ed.) Discussion papers on the pathology of work-related neck and upper limb disorders and the implications for diagnosis and treatment. NCEPH working Paper Number 24, Canberra: National Centre for Epidemiology and Population Health.

Quintner, J.L. and Elvey, R.L. (1993) Understanding 'RSI': a review of the role of peripheral neural pain and hyperalgesia. *J. Manual Manipulative Ther.*, **1**(3), 99–105.

Steindler, A. and Luck, J.V. (1938) Differential diagnosis of pain low in the back. *JAMA*, **110**, 106–13.

Taylor, J.R. and Kakulas, B.A. (1993) Neck injuries. *J. Orthop. Med.*, **15**(1), 10–11.

Travell, J.G. and Simons, D.G. (1983). Myofascial pain and dysfunction. In: *The Trigger Point Manual*. Williams & Wilkins, Baltimore, Md.

Wall, P.D. (1991) Neuropathic pain and injured nerve: central mechanisms. *Br. Med. Bull.*, **47**(3), 631–43.

Wall, P.D. (1994) Introduction to the edition after this one. In *Textbook of Pain* (eds P.D. Wall and R. Melzack), 3rd edn., Churchill Livingstone, Edinburgh, pp. 1–7.

Wigley, R.D., Turner, W.E.D., Blake, B.L. *et al.* (1992) *Occupational Overuse Syndrome. Treatment and Management: A Practitioner's Guide*. Occupational Safety and Health Service, Department of Labour, Wellington, NZ.

Woolf, C.J. (1983) Evidence for a central component of post-injury pain hypersensitivity. *Nature*, **306**, 686–8.

Woolf, C.J. (1991) Generation of acute pain: central mechanisms. *Br. Med. Bull.*, **47**(3), 523–33.

4

Ergonomics

Constant repetition does not seem to induce the state of chronic fatigue so quickly as sustained contraction, because in constantly repeated muscular contraction the muscle enjoys an interval of relaxation and it is in this interval that its nutrition is maintained.

'A telegraphic malady', *Lancet*, 24 April, 1875

Ergonomics is the scientific study of work and is concerned particularly with the design of working systems. It embraces anatomical, biomechanical, psychological and social aspects as far as they relate to the health, safety and performance of the workforce.

The prevention of WRULDs requires critical evaluation of jobs, particularly with respect to matching work (including specific tasks, workplace conditions, equipment and tools) to people's characteristics (McAtamney and Corlett, 1992). Although it is a truism that training and experience are required for people to adapt to work routine, the basic principle underlying good ergonomic practice is to **fit the job and the work-station to the worker**.

Work practices

Poor postures and bad work practices contribute to excessive physiological or biomechanically disadvantageous strains upon tendons at the shoulder, elbow, hand and wrist, upon articular structures (both vertebral and peripheral) and upon the nerves between the spine and the hand. In an extensive review of the literature on ergonomics, Armstrong and colleagues (1987) stated that 'the available data show that hand and wrist tendinitis and related disorders are long-standing causes of worker suffering and lost work in hand intensive industries'. They concluded that there was a 'strong association between the signs and symptoms of hand and wrist tendinitis and *repetitiveness and forcefulness* of manual work'.

In relation to work-related upper limb disorders of all types, ergonomics may be viewed as the study of four key factors: the user, the task, the tool and the environment (personal communication, Andrew Baird, Human Applications, Loughborough, UK). These are summarized as follows:

- **User**
  size (anthropometry)
  shape (for example, the impact of obesity)
  individual susceptibility (for example, carpal tunnel syndrome)
  behaviour (with respect to training, for instance)
  stress
  experience and exposure
- **Task**
  repetition and cycle times
  hours of work
  rest periods
  job rotation
  layout of task (with respect to posture and movements)
  performance requirements (for example, the impact of bonus schemes)
- **Tool**
  posture required
  forces required (for example, grip)
  vibration
  torsion and angulating movements

maintenance (servicing of equipment)

effects of personal protective equipment (for example, gloves)

- **Environment**

physical environment
  - temperature
  - humidity
  - lighting
  - air movements

can have a direct or indirect (behavioural) effect

psychological environment
  - management style
  - peer pressure
  - job satisfaction
  - job security

will affect a person's psychological well-being and their willingness to report problems.

The value of *appropriate training* in many occupations cannot be overemphasized. Musicians who are better trained are less injury-prone: they use their muscles more efficiently and are less likely to produce excessive muscle contractions (Bejjani, 1996).

International perspective

A number of articles in the *Journal of Human Ergology (Tokyo)* in the 1970s and early 1980s reflected the concern about the epidemic of occupational cervicobrachial disorder (OCD), particularly in accounting machine and other keyboard operators, in Japan. The aetiological factors involved in the development of OCD, with particular reference to ergonomics, were studied by the Committee on Occupational Cervicobrachial Syndrome set up by the Japanese Association of Industrial Health. Aoyama *et al.* (1979) reported that the important factors were:

1 dynamic muscle work during repetitive activity;

2 static muscle work, for instance in maintaining elevated arms;

3 muscle overload secondary to adverse posture;

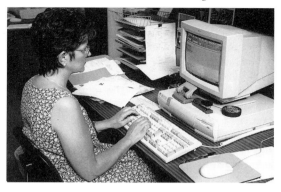

Figure 4.1 Keyboard operators undertake repetitive, high speed movements of the fingers and thumbs

4 mental stress;

5 adverse environmental factors;

6 poor working system design and poor personnel management.

Nakaseko (1982) reviewed the history of OCD in Japan, and commented upon the problems associated with new technology. For instance, it was recognized that VDU operators may make more than 80 000 keystrokes a day (Figure 4.1). It was considered that repetitive, high-speed movements of the fingers, hands and arms were causative factors.

In an oft-quoted study by Silverstein *et al.* (1986) in Michigan, USA, of 574 active workers from six different industrial plants, positive associations were observed between 'hand wrist CTDs' (principally tendon-related disorders and peripheral nerve entrapments) and high force, highly repetitive jobs. The diagnoses were made by structured interview and clinical examination. Videotape recordings and EMG studies were used to estimate hand force and repetitiveness. The findings were similar to other studies, the overall prevalence in women being 13.6%.

Neck and upper limb symptoms were recorded by Maeda *et al.* (1980) in Swiss accounting machine operators in whom there was an identifiable *static* load on the postural muscles of the neck and shoulder region as well as a combination of static and dynamic loads on the arm and hand muscles. The importance of static loading of the muscles of the neck–shoulder region, often associated with persistently poor posture during work activities, particularly at a keyboard, has been stressed by many authors.

McDermott (1986) reviewed the contemporaneous understanding of 'repetition strain injury', and referred to the contribution of ergonomic factors to the epidemic of RSI in Australia in the 1980s. A wide spectrum of adverse ergonomic factors was noted, including inappropriate viewing angles and poor work-station layout for VDU operators. The muscle activities that were associated with RSI in one study were static muscle load with abduction of the shoulders, the hand pinch grip, and the hand grasp grip. Many workers in light industry, as well as keyboard operators, held their wrists in ulnar deviation (Figure 4.2); however, it should be noted that slight extension and ulnar deviation of the wrist is the optimal position for hand function (Tubiana and Chamagne, 1988). Work stress, for instance excessive noise, work quota deadlines, inadequate rest breaks and a conflict between monotony and concentration were acknowledged as contributory factors. Work strain has been accorded important aetiological status by many authors, although its relationship to premorbid personality traits is often anecdotal or speculative.

Hocking (1987) reflected upon the possible contribution of ergonomic factors in the epidemic of RSI in Telecom Australia. The diagnosis of RSI was based on accident reports and medical certificates, incorporating both

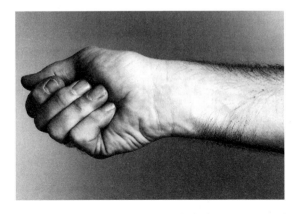

Figure 4.2 Ulnar deviation and slight extension of the wrist is the optimal position for hand function.

type 1 and type 2 WRULD. A rate of 343 per 1000 telephonists with RSI over the five-year period 1981–5 contrasted with a rate of 34 per 1000 telegraphists. This contrasting incidence in the two groups was the inverse of the keystroke rate (a few hundred an hour for telephonists and over 12 000 an hour for telegraphists), prompting Hocking to opine that the keystroke rate, which had previously (and subsequently) been considered to be a contributory factor, played little part in the aetiology of 'RSI'.

In addition to the lack of a consistent dose–response relationship between keystroke rate and occupational groupings of RSI, Hocking found little relationship to age and job duration too. He advised caution when predicting health consequences (in the form of type 2 WRULD) from simple ergonomic assessments of work-stations, stating that '**the mere finding of ergonomic problems does not prove that they are directly causal of – or even predisposing factors to – "RSI"** '.

When analysing the role of psychosocial factors as well as adverse ergonomics in RSI, Hocking noted that there was a considerable geographical variation in the distribution of cases of RSI in telephone staff members among states. The lowest incidence of RSI occurred in New South Wales, in spite of its work-stress problems (for instance, poor job satisfaction) noted by other workers. Interestingly, in a review of the incidence of cases of RSI at Telecom Australia two years later, Hocking (1989) also opined that there was no evidence for the view that secondary gain might have caused the 'epidemic'. The marked decline in the number of cases (from 1985 onwards) took place well before the court judgments that failed to uphold common law claims.

There was also a significant geographical variation in the incidence of RSI in data processing operators who were employed by the Australian Bureau of Statistics (McDermott, 1986). Whilst the overall incidence of new cases rose from 2% in 1975–6 to 11% in 1981–2 the increase was dramatic in New South Wales, Victoria and the Australian Capital Territory, but the incidence remained low and virtually unaltered in Queensland, Western Australia and Tasmania. For this and other reasons, the need for carefully designed epidemiological studies of work-related upper limb disorders is paramount.

Identification of adverse workplace environmental factors

Complex situations usually demand appropriate training of in-house personnel with ergonomic consultancy support. For the less complex situation, trained staff may be recommended to use Appendix 2 ('A checklist for the identification and reduction of work-related upper limb disorders') of the HSE booklet *Work Related Upper Limb Disorders* (1990) as a resource in identifying adverse ergonomic factors that are often interacting. The relevant questions that should be asked include the following.

- **Personal**
  (a) Has the training programme addressed an individual's requirements? Has everything been done to reduce boredom and anxiety, and to maximize relaxation and coordination?
  (b) Are efforts continually made by supervisory staff to reduce workplace tensions, and to collaborate regarding improvements in the work process? Are management's demands stressful? Is the general environment a source of discontent?
  (c) Have anthropometric factors been taken into account? Have adequate steps been taken to accommodate the job to the worker?
- **Work activity**
  (a) Is the tool size appropriate to the job and to the individual? Do the tool or machinery handles comply with ergonomic criteria?
  (b) Are forces applied close to the extremes of joint movement? Is repetition kept to a minimum?
  (c) Are the arms held at mechanically disadvantageous positions (particularly when raised high or away from the body)? Do the work activities allow maintenance of the natural spinal curves?

(d) Have the effects of vibration been minimized, for example by vibration absorbing grips?
(e) Have appropriate tool design measures been undertaken to reduce the need for relatively stressful grips such as the pinch grip in favour of the power grip?
(f) Has the work-station layout been critically evaluated, particularly with respect to each individual worker?
(g) Does the work activity include frequent short rest periods? Is job rotation available?

Muscular 'work'

Occupational activities in general require a combination of isotonic and isometric contraction. Professional musicians, particularly violinists (see Figure 1.4), are a typical example of an occupational group in whom isotonic contractions in fingers and wrists are combined with isometric loading of the muscles of the shoulder girdle.

Movement results from isotonic contraction, either concentric or eccentric, the resultant work (in ergonomic terms) being referred to sometimes as 'dynamic work'. Despite its often repetitive nature, dynamic work may be maintained for a longer period of time prior to the onset of fatigue than 'static work' in which isometric contraction is the principal component. Static work is at the core of many manual activities in which gripping is a feature (Figure 4.3). Postural muscles, for instance the scapular fixators, undergo static contraction too (Figure 4.4); when postural loading is unusually high, particularly when working in cramped or constrained postures, fatigue occurs relatively quickly.

As most ergonomists presume that the *early* stages of type 2 WRULD are caused by a combination of *excessively prolonged static muscle tension* and 'stress', the importance of sound ergonomic principles cannot be overstated. Clearly, there is individual variation in physiological tolerance to static muscle loading, and training may play a considerable role. Equally important is individual susceptibility to environmental stresses (sometimes referred

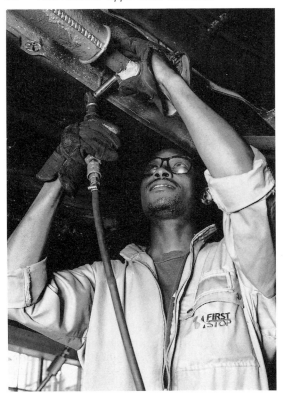

Figure 4.3 Repetitive or sustained elevation of the arms at shoulder height and above is a recognized stressor for the rotator cuff

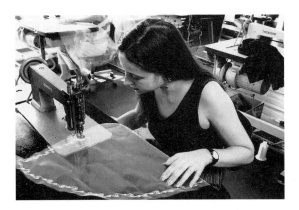

Figure 4.4 Discomfort in the neck and shoulders is virtually endemic in sewing machinists

to as 'stress reactivity'). The development of type 2 WRULD would appear to be related to *the way* in which the susceptible person interacts with their environment when subject to

discomfort from soft tissue nociceptive stimulation (Darby and Brown, 1990). As a corollary, management of muscle tension pain should be by **relaxation** and **stress management training**.

Logistics

The Health and Safety at Work Act 1974 placed a duty upon employers to ensure, as far as is reasonably practicable, the health, safety and welfare at work of all their employees. The Management of Health and Safety at Work Regulations 1992 generally make more explicit the requirements of employers under the Act, for instance the need to carry out risk assessments, across the full range of workplaces. More specific requirements are identified in other Regulations: work-stations and seating are included in the Workplace (Health, Safety and Welfare) Regulations 1992; lifting and handling are encompassed by the Manual Handling Operations Regulations 1992; the requirements for visual display units are set out in the Health and Safety (Display Screen Equipment) Regulations 1992 – otherwise known as the VDU Regulations. The VDU Regulations came into force in the UK on 1 January 1993, putting into UK law a European Community Directive to reduce the following health risks:

1   upper limb disorder (including pains in the neck, arms, elbows, wrists, hands, fingers);
2   temporary eyestrain and headaches;
3   fatigue and stress.

Although assistance may be required by employers from ergonomists or forensic engineers in identifying inadequate work practices, little difficulty should be experienced by any health professional (engaged in occupational health work) in identifying poor work postures. The Health and Safety Executive publications in the UK, and equivalent publications abroad, amply demonstrate the methodology for risk assessment and for the identification and reduction of work-related upper limb disorders. Postural problems in keyboard operators were addressed by Grandjean in his seminal work, 'Ergonomics and health in modern offices' (1984). Since then, guidelines for the optimal work-station

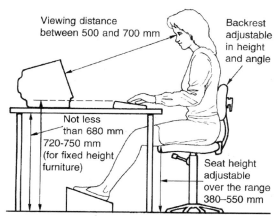

Viewing distance between 500 and 700 mm

Backrest adjustable in height and angle

Not less than 680 mm
720-750 mm (for fixed height furniture)

Seat height adjustable over the range 380–550 mm

The surface area of the desk is large enough to accommodate all necessary equipment and documents required for the task, in the correct positions

Unobstructed area beneath desk is
Width   800 mm
Depth   750 mm (foot level)
            500 mm (knee level)

Figure 4.5 An example of guidelines for the optimal dimensions of the keyboard operative's workstation

dimensions have become readily available (Figure 4.5).

Postural training is a particularly important issue for those engaged in prolonged sitting. Good cervicodorsal posture is dependent upon maintenance of the lumbar lordosis. Chair modifications to prevent the loss of the lumbar lordosis include a built-in adjustable lumbar support, a facility to increase the forward slope of the seat, and measures to raise or lower the height of the seat from the floor (Figure 4.6). Ergonomic attention to the height of the work surface when handwriting, drawing or studying is also helpful in maintaining the cervical lordosis (Figure 4.7). It is conceivable that future changes in work-station design will include the facility for optional sit–stand operation by the provision of hydraulically adjustable desk tops.

Summary

McPhee (1987) has categorized ergonomic factors into the following groups from which potential stressors may be identified as contributors to WRULDs, particularly when several are present concurrently causing cumulative stress.

1 **External factors**
    number of movements;
    static muscle work;
    force;
    work postures determined by the equipment and furniture;
    time worked without a break.
2 **Factors which influence the load but which may vary between individuals**
    work posture adopted;
    unnecessary use of force or static muscle work;
    need for speed and accuracy of movements;
    frequency and duration of pauses taken by the operator.
3 **Factors which alter the individual's response to a particular load**
    individual factors (experience, training, anthropometry, age, fitness);

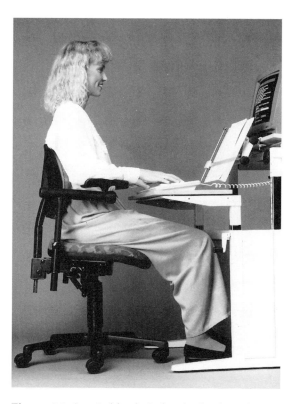

Figure 4.6 A suitable chair for the keyboard operator is demonstrated. (Courtesy of Advance Seating Designs)

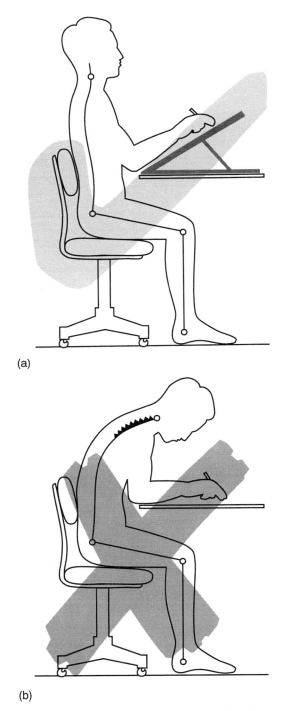

(a)

(b)

Figure 4.7 Maintenance of the cervical lordosis is assisted by this Posturite work-top board: (*a*, *b*) diagrammatic representation (courtesy of A-Design Limited); (*c*) in practice

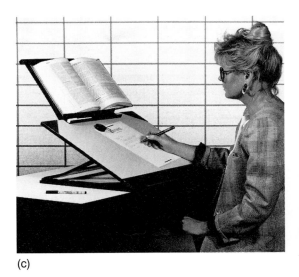

(c)

workplace environmental factors (lighting, thermal climate, noise, vibration);
psychosocial variables.

In short, special attention should be paid to the following physical stress factors:

- the force exerted (in relation to the capacity of the muscles);
- awkward posture (with respect to the upper limbs and the body weight);
- repetitive activities;
- rest periods – duration and frequency;

and to the following individual susceptibility to stress:

- physiological vulnerability;
- psychological vulnerability.

Type 1 WRULDs may be prevented by good ergonomic design of tools, workplaces and equipment, good job design and good organizational arrangements such as training, job rotation and work organization. The prevention of type 2 WRULD is more complex, and the effectiveness of traditional ergonomics techniques is questionable. Psychological factors such as job satisfaction probably play as important a role as work-station design.

References

Aoyama, H., Ohara, H., Oze, Y. and Itani, T. (1979) Recent trends in research on occupational cervicobrachial disorder. *J. Human Ergol. (Tokyo)*, **8**, 39–45.

Armstrong, T.J., Fine, L.J., Goldstein, S.A. Lifshitz, Y.R. and Silverstein, B.A. (1987) Ergonomics considerations in hand and wrist tendinitis. *J. Hand Surg.*, **12A**(5), 830–7.

Bejjani, F.J., Kaye G.M. and Benham, M. (1996) Musculoskeletal and neuromuscular conditions of instrumental musicians. *Arch. Phys. Med. Rehabil.*, **77**, 406–13.

Darby, F.W. and Brown, D.A. (1990) On site management of occupational overuse and fatigue. A training workshop in practical skills. Occupational Health Task Force, Department of Health, NZ.

Grandjean, E. (1984) Postural problems at office machine work stations. In: *Ergonomics and Health in Modern Offices* (ed. E. Grandjean), Taylor and Francis, London.

Hocking, B. (1987) Epidemiological aspects of 'repetition strain injury' in Telecom Australia. *Med. J. Aust.*, **147**, 218–22.

Hocking, B. (1989) 'Repetition strain injury' in Telecom Australia. *Med. J. Aust.*, **150**, 724.

McAtamney, L. and Corlett, E.N. (1992) Reducing the risks of work related upper limb disorders. A guide and methods. Institute for Occupational Ergonomics, University of Nottingham.

McDermott, F.T. (1986) Repetition strain injury: a review of current understanding. *Med. J. Aust.*, **144**, 196–200.

McPhee, B.J. (1987) Work-related musculoskeletal disorders of the neck and upper extremities in workers engaged in light, highly repetitive work. In: *Proceedings of an International Symposium: Work-Related Musculoskeletal Disorders* (eds U. Osterholz, W. Karmaus, B. Hullman and B. Ritz), Bonn, pp. 244–58.

Maeda, K., Hunting, W. and Grandjean, E. (1980) Localised fatigue in accounting-machine operators. *J. Occup. Med.*, **22**(12), 810–16.

Nakaseko, M., Tokunaga, R. and Hosokawa, M. (1982) History of occupational cervicobrachial disorder in Japan. *J. Human Ergol. (Tokyo)*, **11**, 7–16.

Silverstein, B.A., Fine, L.J. and Armstrong, T.J. (1986) Hand wrist cumulative trauma disorders in industry. *Br. J. Industr. Med.*, **43**, 779–84.

Tubiana, R. and Chamagne, P. (1988) Functional anatomy of the hand. *Med. Probl. Performing Artists*, September, pp. 83–7.

Work-related Upper Limb Disorders. A Guide to Prevention (1990) Health and Safety Executive, HSE Books, Suffolk, UK.

5

Type 1 WRULDs

Disease is very old, and nothing about it has changed. It is we who change, as we learn to recognize what was formerly imperceptible.

Jean Martin Charcot (1825–93), 'De l'expectation en médecine'

In the workplace, as elsewhere, neuromuscular reflex activity is an automatic and subconscious response to biomechanical stresses in an attempt to maintain postural equilibrium (Kuchera, 1995). When the adaptive viscoelastic (deformation) properties of the connective tissues are overwhelmed by physical forces, including the static and dynamic stresses of the workplace, musculoskeletal strains occur.

I have chosen to label the soft tissue and neural conditions described in this chapter type 1 work-related upper limb disorders (type 1 WRULDs). They constitute the commonly accepted overuse conditions affecting the upper limbs such as rotator cuff tendinitis, tennis elbow and golfer's elbow, tenosynovitis and tenovaginitis, and peripheral nerve entrapment.

These are ubiquitous conditions that conform to 'disease' in the conventional disease-illness model. They have clearly defined and distinguishable subjective symptoms (Ireland, 1988) and clinical signs that are reliably reproducible. There are demonstrable morphological changes and appropriate treatment strategies. It should be noted however that a cause and effect relationship between occupation and type 1 WRULDs may not always be present in individual patients: it is incumbent upon the clinician to evaluate the various stressors in each case.

The differential diagnosis in this heterogeneous group of overuse conditions must always be referred phenomena, from the neck particularly. Accordingly, an account of somatic dysfunction affecting the cervicothoracic spine, which may also play a part in the development of the regional pain syndrome (type 2 WRULD) described in Chapter 6, is included in this chapter.

ENTHESOPATHIES

The entheses are the insertions of collagenous structures such as tendons, ligaments and articular capsules into bone. The morphological characteristics of an enthesis include the attachment portion of the tendon, the attachment portion of the bone (which is not covered by periosteum) and interposed hyaline cartilage; the paratenon merges with the periosteum. The layer of cartilage adjacent to bone is calcified and merges without a defined border into the bony structure (Niepel and Sit'aj, 1979).

Physiologically, the entheses are subjected to immense loads, but it is probably repeated stresses that cause the characteristic changes of enthesitis (or 'enthesopathy'). The entheses are relatively avascular, and therefore vulnerable to repetitive traction. Enthesopathies are usually localized to one specific area, but they may arise as part of the systemic manifestation of inflammatory rheumatic disorders; they may also be relatively generalized in a subgroup of the population that is prone to 'non-articular rheumatism' and in whom metabolic and endocrine factors may play an important role. Examples of commonly recognized enthesopathies are insertional supraspinatus tendinitis, adductor longus tendinitis and plantar fasciitis. This chapter will confine discussion to lateral epicondylitis and medial epicondylitis.

Lateral epicondylitis

Epidemiology and aetiology

The terms lateral epicondylitis and tennis elbow are used synonymously in this text. According to Boyd and McLeod (1973) the condition was first described by Runge (100 years previously, in 1873). However, Golding (1986) noted a description by Renton in 1830 in which the described management of 'a painful affection of the supinator radii longus' was by acupuncture. Cyriax (1936) cites Morris (1882) who called it 'lawn-tennis arm' and noted its similarity to rider's sprain. Major (1883) and Winckworth (1883) may have been responsible for coining the term (lawn) 'tennis elbow'.

Lateral epicondylitis is one of the most common soft tissue lesions of the arm. It affects 1% of manual workers (Kivi, 1982), usually occurring in the dominant arm. It is rare under the age of 30. Tennis players constitute a significant, if minority, group of sufferers.

Gruchow and Pelletier (1979) noted an incidence of 39.7% in more than 500 tennis players (Figure 5.1). In my view, a technical fault on the backhand, usually a jerky shot with backspin, is responsible for the onset of the condition. The use of the modern racquet (graphite, for instance), which does not absorb vibrations as well as the 'old-fashioned' wooden racquet, may be another factor in some cases. Although patients may recall the occasion, or indeed the shot, when pain was first experienced, it is probable that in the vast majority of cases this constitutes the final stage of a gradual loss of adaptation to repetitive stresses imposed upon the common extensor origin. In other words, the condition is an overuse injury.

In the workplace lateral epicondylitis arises as a result of repetitive grasping, the use of pinch movements, or the power grip – usually in 'blue-collar' workers (see Figure 7.31). The common factor could be the stabilization of the wrist (by concurrent extensor and flexor contraction) to allow the repetitive or forceful hand movements. The aetiological stresses often include frequent forceful supination but the primary stressor is repetitive firm grasping which is an action that is required of some workers many thousand times daily. Kivi judged that 73% of cases (64 from 88) of lateral

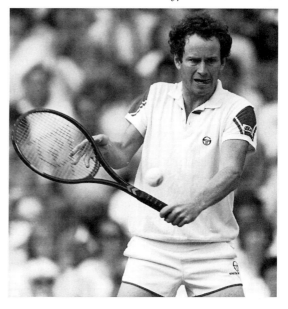

Figure 5.1 The backhand tennis shot imposes considerable strain upon the wrist dorsiflexors. (Courtesy of Bob Thomas)

epicondylitis in manual workers were occupational; 27% resulted from spare-time activity.

The relatively high incidence in some series of lateral epicondylitis in females between the ages of 40 and 60 years is probably due to the lower resilience of tendons, and in particular teno-osseous junctions, to repeated biomechanical stresses in middle age (at a time when socioeconomic pressures often demand maximization of family income).

It is generally undisputed that housewives, irrespective of whether or not they are also in full-time remunerative employment, engage in just those activities – carrying heavy shopping baskets, cleaning, general housework and cooking – that demand repeated grasping, often firm and prolonged grasping. Middle-aged females (and, in the modern era of the 'new man', middle-aged males too who contribute to general household and DIY activities) may be considered to be particularly vulnerable when engaged in two occupations – domestic and industrial – that are excessively demanding of their elbow entheses. With respect to the relationship between elbow pain and work, prospective employers should be aware of the vulnerability of the 'middle-aged'.

The epidemiological evidence to support the causal association between work activity and tennis elbow is far from conclusive. Kivi (1982) considered that overexertion of the finger and wrist extensors in manual workers was the cause of lateral epicondylitis in a high percentage of cases. Gellman (1992) opined that there is a definite association, for instance with occupations such as carpentry (with which I concur). Electricians and fitters are a vulnerable group as a result of the repeated use of pliers of different types (Kurppa *et al.*, 1979). Other researchers have been unable to find any evidence for increased incidence in manual workers, or even in females. Wadsworth (1987) finds it more common in men. Regrettably, the available data are often composed of small study numbers and are affected by poor study design.

Pathoanatomy

Lateral epicondylitis is a typical example of an enthesopathy, in which microtears of the tendon are associated with disruption of the zone of calcification at the teno-osseous junction (Figure 5.2). In advanced cases small portions of bone and cartilage may become separated. During the repair process well-vascularized granulation tissue is seen; calcification of collagen fibres and formation of new bone may occur.

Goldie (1964) described pathological changes in the soft tissues around the lateral epicondyle. Coonrad and Hooper (1973) noted gross pathological changes, including tears, in the affected tendons in both medial and lateral epicondylitis. A common finding is mesenchymal transformation, calcification and new bone formation (Chard and Hazleman, 1989). Nirschl (1986) has described the microscopic appearances as 'angiofibroblastic hyperplasia'; at surgery the affected area of the common extensor tendon may reveal a somewhat oedematous, greyish tissue.

The pathological changes are caused by repetitive and cumulative overload, though occasionally preceding direct trauma is reported. Although, as previously noted, many tennis elbow specimens show degenerative changes, **the primary cause is essentially microtraumatic**. In some patients a more profound tear of the affected tendon origin is seen at surgery.

The tendon most frequently affected is extensor carpi radialis brevis (ECRB). Its origin is the lateral epicondyle which is the site of maximal tenderness in the vast majority of patients, as opposed to the supracondylar ridge from whence extensor carpi radialis longus (ECRL) originates (Figure 5.3). The distinction from extensor digitorum is suggested by the increased pain on isometric wrist dorsiflexion when resistance is applied by the examiner to the dorsum of the metacarpals rather than to the dorsum of the fingers.

Clinical features

Lateral epicondylitis is characterized by lateral elbow discomfort, sometimes radiating to the extensor aspect of the forearm, but rarely associated with discomfort proximal to the elbow. A more widespread distribution of symptoms, particularly when associated with discomfort in the neck and shoulder or in the medial aspect of the ipsilateral elbow or in the contralateral elbow, suggests alternative pathology – possibly neuropathic arm pain, cervical spinal joint dysfunction or fibromyalgia. A common complaint is 'weakness' of grip. Further enquiry reveals that attempts to grip hard are accompanied by pain.

Commonly, the discomfort associated with lateral epicondylitis worsens, the condition behaving as a typical overuse syndrome. Over a period of some weeks patients usually find that all activities that necessitate gripping or pinching become painful. Holding a cup by applying a pinch grip to the handle is often painful. The symptoms are activity-dependent, resolving at rest and not disturbing sleep.

Paraesthesiae and numbness are not features of lateral epicondylitis. Their presence in the hand raises the possibility of entrapment neuropathy – for instance in the neck, very occasionally in the proximal forearm (for instance, the superficial radial nerve) or at the wrist. Paraesthesiae and hyperalgesia are also features of neuropathic arm pain.

Examination findings

The examination findings in the typical case leave little room for doubt about the diagnosis. In the more severe form, there is soft tissue swelling (oedema) overlying the lateral

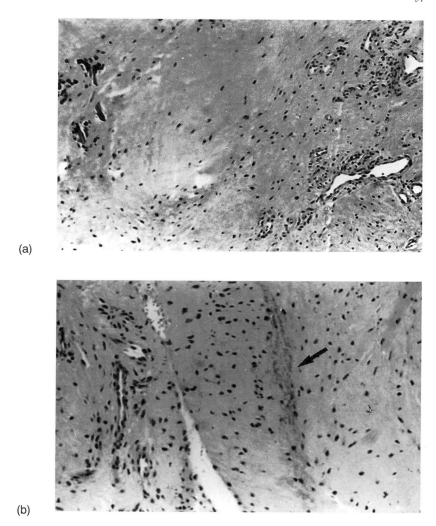

(a)

(b)

Figure 5.2 The typical histopathological findings in lateral epicondylitis of the elbow are illustrated in these specimens of excised tendinous insertion: (*a*) microcalcification and increased vascularity; (*b*) hyper-vascularity, scanty perivascular lymphocytic infiltrate, and myxoid degeneration of tendon collagen (*arrow*). (Courtesy of A. Stevens, Department of Histopathology, University Hospital, Nottingham)

epicondyle. There may be a springy block to full extension (a confounding feature unless one postulates an associated localized inflammatory reaction affecting the adjacent synovial lining of the capitello-radial joint); however, flexion of the elbow is invariably of full painless range. This distinguishes the condition from a lesion affecting the radiohumeral joint, such as osteoarthritis. Full painless extension is soon regained as the condition resolves.

The combination of palmarflexion of the wrist, pronation of the forearm and extension of the elbow provokes discomfort (by stretching the affected tendon). This is sometimes referred to as Mills' test (see Figure 7.19).

The standard finding is pain on resisted contraction of the wrist dorsiflexors – particularly when resisting dorsiflexion of the wrist with fingers semiflexed. Resisted extension of the fingers and resisted radial deviation of the wrist are painful to lesser degrees.

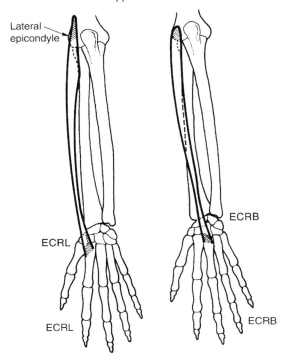

Lateral epicondyle

ECRB

ECRL

ECRL

ECRB

Figure 5.3 The extensores carpi radialis (ECRL and ECRB)

Resisted supination is not usually painful. (Should resisted supination provoke discomfort, posterior interosseous nerve entrapment should be considered in the differential diagnosis.)

Tenderness is localized to the anterior margin of the lateral epicondyle, at the origin of ECRB, in the vast majority of cases. Tenderness may be felt in atypical cases along the supracondylar ridge, at the orbicular ligament, or in the common extensor muscle bellies approximately 6 cm distal to the lateral epicondyle. Tenderness at any site is often exquisite but should nevertheless be assessed by comparison with the non-painful limb.

Investigations are unnecessary in the straightforward case. Occasionally radiography is helpful to exclude arthritis. Serological investigation for conditions such as gout or a rheumatic diathesis may be necessary in the presence of more generalized symptoms or signs.

Management

Cyriax (1969) advised that, if left untreated (and presumably rested from provocative activity initially), the natural outcome is for spontaneous resolution over the course of approximately 12 months. Understandably, whether the condition arises through sport or as a result of overuse at home or at work, most patients seek treatment for their pain. If offered the options of active treatment or prolonged rest most will request a management strategy that will attempt to foreshorten the period of disability.

A reasonable assumption might be that anti-inflammatory measures in the form of physiotherapy (for instance cryotherapy or ultrasound) and pharmaceutical preparations (for instance NSAIDs) should be effective. However, it is a common experience that none of the aforementioned therapies offers more than minimal benefit. If combined with rest, it is more likely to be the rest that is most effective.

The amount of rest depends on the severity of the condition. A reduction in work intensity or a change in activity may be effective. A modification of sports technique may be helpful. (This certainly applies to racquet-players' lateral epicondylitis.) In the established case complete rest from provocative activities (indicating the need for some time off work) is necessary. These are the circumstances in which a localized steroid injection is most effective. Conversely, a common therapeutic error is to allow patients to work more or less straight away after an injection, thereby failing to maximize the effectiveness of the treatment.

A *maximum* dosage for a long-acting steroid should be 10 mg triamcinolone acetonide (for instance, 1 ml Adcortyl) or 25 mg hydrocortisone (for instance, 1 ml Hydrocortistab). A very common mistake is to overdose – for instance, to use 1 ml of preparations such as Kenalog (40 mg triamcinolone hexacetonide) or Depomedrone (40 mg methyl prednisolone) – when the likelihood of unwelcome skin and subcutaneous side effects (pallor, telangiectasia and atrophy of subcutaneous fat) is significantly raised.

As with all injection treatments for enthesopathies, the injection should be given in droplet form (but with a single skin penetration) to the teno-osseous junction: the end of the needle should abut bone. An equal volume of local anaesthetic may be used as this gives

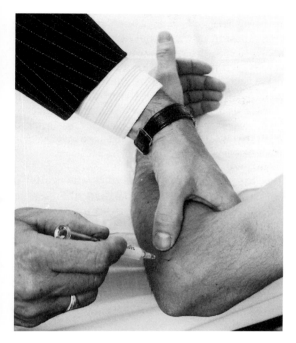

Figure 5.4 The patient sits with the elbow in 90 degrees flexion for injection of lateral epicondylitis

very rapid relief of symptoms to the satisfaction of the patient and the doctor (Figure 5.4).

My practice is to inject 2 ml of solution – 1 ml Adcortyl and 1 ml 1% lignocaine – using a 2 ml syringe and a 23 gauge needle. If the diagnosis is correct, the injection is initially painful, then painless within a minute or two as the local anaesthetic takes effect. Patients should be warned of the likelihood of increased discomfort for 24 hours, following which they are often asymptomatic (or much improved) within a few days. However, there is a risk of incomplete healing unless a minimum period of 2–3 weeks is allowed for the healing process to be consolidated. In this sense a comparison may be made with the healing of a fracture: it is not until the healing has progressed from the stage when the fracture has united to the consolidation stage that the affected site may be subjected safely to 'normal' stresses.

If the subject is still symptomatic, or if resisted contraction of extensor carpi radialis is still painful, after 2–3 weeks, the injection should be repeated. As before, 5–10 mg of triamcinolone should be used. Treatment may be considered to be complete when the subject no longer experiences pain when the previously provocative tasks are undertaken and when the clinical signs are also negative. Slight epicondylar tenderness may be accepted if this is the only abnormal sign.

Physiotherapeutic modalities are often helpful in those sufferers who experience significant tenderness and discomfort from the common extensor muscle belly in the forearm in addition to (or in lieu of) tenderness at the lateral epicondyle. Transverse friction massage is the preferred treatment at this site.

Recurrent tennis elbow is as difficult to treat as the majority of tennis elbows are easy. If pain recurs within a few months of its initial successful management, the likelihood of a satisfactory outcome with further injections is significantly reduced. An analysis of the level of activities undertaken – at work, domestic and recreational – will usually identify the major stressors. A more radical assessment of the aetiological factors – the type of activity, its frequency and intensity, and the frequency of rest periods for instance – will be required.

The use of an epicondylitis clasp is found to be helpful by some patients. Its mode of action is far from clear; amelioration of symptoms may be the result of neurophysiological suppression of pain perception (by mechanoreceptor stimulus) rather than by reduction of biomechanical stress at the epicondyle (following modification of forearm rotation, for instance).

Patients with recalcitrant tennis elbow may be treated by localized sclerosant injections (of 25% dextrose and 2% phenol), by surgery (Nirschl and Pettrone, 1979), or by a Mills' manipulation under general anaesthetic. A tendon slide under local anaesthetic is the simplest and possibly the most effective surgical procedure. Wadsworth (1987) has reported good results with a Mills' manipulation (forceful extension of the elbow with the forearm pronated and the wrist palmarflexed – after Mills, 1928). It is doubtful whether any of these methods should be viewed prospectively as sufficiently reliable for patients to contemplate a return to unrestricted manual activity in the future. In my own experience of sclerosant injections, the results may be gratifying after years of discomfort.

Outcome

Although most patients respond to the combination of a low dose steroid injection and a period of rest, relapse of the condition within a few months is associated with a much reduced likelihood of complete resolution with further injections. There is anecdotal evidence that the condition is likely to persist well beyond one year following failed steroid injections. However, cause and effect are not established as this may equally well constitute a subgroup of patients with recalcitrant lesions, whatever the management strategy.

Some particularly susceptible individuals continue to experience symptoms from lateral epicondylitis recurrently for many years. However, most sufferers find that their symptoms resolve eventually – often within 12–18 months – but this is dependent upon whether reduction of provocative stress has been possible. Should a manual worker change to another job or another occupation that is as demanding of the muscles of grip and grasp as before, it is likely that symptoms from tennis elbow will continue *ad infinitum*. The natural history of the condition and the need for a moderation of work activity indicate that the sufferer is disadvantaged in an open labour market for at least one or two years.

Failure to achieve a temporary respite of symptoms raises the question of inexpert injection technique or misdiagnosis. In the framework of work-relatedness, misdiagnosis usually results from the failure to recognize the condition of neuropathic arm pain, in which hyperalgesia in the region of the common extensor origin is a marked feature in the majority of patients. Examination of the neck and arm for evidence of neural tension or features of neurosensitization is mandatory in patients with elbow pain.

Very occasionally, the radial tunnel syndrome is encountered. The radial tunnel runs from the head of the radius to the supinator muscle. Roles and Maudsley (1972) considered that resistant cases of tennis elbow are explained on the basis of entrapment neuropathy of the radial nerve and/or its branches. They supported their hypothesis in a series of cases by successful surgical release of the entrapment through an anterior muscle-splitting incision. It has been postulated that compression of the radial nerve, or the nerves (posterior interosseous and superficial radial) into which it divides is more likely in occupations in which there is frequent forceful supination and pronation of the arm.

Medial epicondylitis

Aetiology

The terms medial epicondylitis and golfer's elbow are used synonymously in this text.

Right-handed golfers may experience medial epicondylitis of their right elbow if they have a 'strong right hand' (that is, if there is excessive pronation of the forearm during uncocking of the wrist at ball strike). This observation is of considerable importance aetiologically as it is likely that repeated forceful pronation of the forearm is the cause of medial epicondylitis in the majority of cases. This is supported by the observation of Nirschl (1986) that pathological changes are found in the origin of pronator teres and flexor carpi radialis from the medial epicondyle (Figure 5.5).

Medial epicondylitis is probably most common in middle-aged women, but statistics are hard to come by. I eschew the fatalistic approach that considers that the condition is 'constitutional', inferring that it is inevitable in a section of the population. Various activities around the house, in the garden, or in the home workshop may provoke its onset. Tennis players with a wristy forehand are a vulnerable group. In the workplace, repetitive forceful pronation is the usual stressor.

Clinical features

Discomfort is experienced at the medial epicondyle and along the volar aspect of the forearm. Rarely is the discomfort as severe as that experienced in lateral epicondylitis, nor the dysfunction as profound. Paraesthesiae are not experienced; differentiation from the pronator syndrome is necessary if sensory symptoms are experienced distally in the median nerve distribution.

In common with lateral epicondylitis the symptoms improve with rest but recur with repetitive grasping and, particularly, with repetitive pronation of the forearm. Medial epicondylitis usually resolves spontaneously

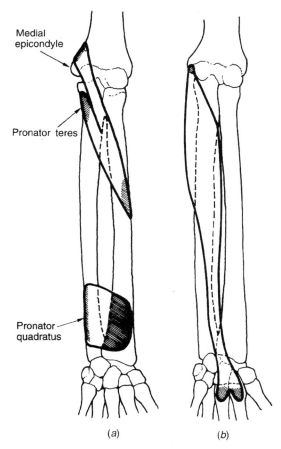

Medial
epicondyle

Pronator teres

Pronator
quadratus

(a)   (b)

Figure 5.5 Pathological changes are found in the origin of (*a*) pronator teres and (*b*) flexor carpi radialis, from the medial epicondyle in 'golfer's elbow'. The attachments of these muscles are illustrated

over somewhat longer than 12 months if the stresses applied to the elbow are reduced.

Examination findings

In the uncomplicated case there are no abnormalities of the cervical spine, and no evidence of nerve root entrapment or peripheral nerve entrapment. The movements of the elbow joint are of full range. The combination of passive dorsiflexion of the wrist, supination of the forearm and extension of the elbow provokes medial elbow discomfort. Pain on resisted pronation of the forearm is the most reliable sign on the isometric contraction tests.

Discomfort on resisted wrist flexion is not always present.

Tenderness is localized to the common flexor origin, approximately 1 cm distal to the tip of the medial epicondyle. It is unusual for tenderness to be detected elsewhere; if present in the bulk of muscles in the volar aspect of the forearm several centimetres from the elbow, careful assessment for more generalized hyperalgesia must be made.

Although the ulnar nerve in its cubital tunnel is in close proximity to the common flexor origin from the medial epicondyle, it is positioned posteriorly and is not subject to compression or irritation by medial epicondylitis. In the pronator syndrome neuritic symptoms are present and weakness may be detected on resisted pronation of the forearm, resisted finger flexion and resisted opposition of the thumb.

Management

In principle, management is along similar lines as for lateral epicondylitis. Appropriate measures should be undertaken to reduce overload at the common flexor origin. A change of work routine may suffice in the early or non-severe case. In the established case a period off work may be necessary. Under these circumstances (that is, when a period of rest is prescribed) a clinical decision should be made as to whether to treat by localized steroid injection. If the diagnosis is correct, an injection of 10 mg triamcinolone or equivalent successfully abolishes discomfort within a few days; usually there is good correlation between improvement in the clinical signs and subjective improvement. A further injection may be required after 3 weeks if symptoms persist, albeit at a reduced intensity.

Provided that the site of tenderness on the volar aspect of the medial epicondyle is positively identified, there is no danger of damage to the ulnar nerve. However, I have encountered an occasional case of apparent increased sensitivity of the ulnar nerve, possibly as a result of aberrant anatomical position, resulting in transient paraesthesiae in the distal ulnar distribution following injection of golfer's elbow. The responsiveness of medial epicondylitis to conventional physiotherapeutic anti-inflammatory measures is similar to that of lateral epicondylitis – modest at best.

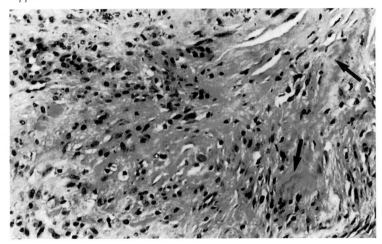

Figure 5.6 The typical histopathological features of de Quervain's tenovaginitis are demonstrated. This biopsied thickened tendon sheath reveals hypervascularity, scanty perivascular lymphocytic infiltrate and increased numbers of plump active fibroblasts. There is focal myxoid degeneration of collagen (*arrows*). (Courtesy of A. Stevens, Department of Histopathology, University Hospital, Nottingham)

Outcome

This is dependent upon a number of variables, including adequate reduction of overload at the elbow, appropriate treatment and correct diagnosis. The following are some of the features that suggest that the diagnosis of lateral or medial epicondylitis may be *incorrect*.

1 Generalized hyperalgesia.
2 Hyperalgesia in the absence of pain on resisted muscle contraction.
3 Bilateral symptoms.
4 Concomitant lateral and medial epicondylitis affecting the same elbow.
5 The presence of paraesthesiae and/or numbness distally.
6 Failure to respond to local steroid injection.

TENDINOPATHIES

General considerations

Tendinopathies in the hand, wrist and forearm are common conditions. Although they are frequently transient they may assume a chronic state, severely compromising the ability to work. Despite the arguments regarding nomenclature and, in particular, the lack of histopathological evidence to support an inflammatory basis in many instances, these

conditions are frequently the result of *overuse*. As such, occupational factors should always be considered amongst other aetiological stressors.

The conventional view of tendinitis (more appropriately termed *tendinosis*) is that collagen fibril microfailure arises as a result of repetitive, and finally excessive, demands on a tendon. When a tendon is covered by a paratenon a secondary inflammatory reaction gives rise to paratendinitis, as in paratendinitis crepitans (intersection syndrome). When tendons run through fibro-osseous channels, for instance at the wrist, they have a lining (teno)synovium as well as a fibrous sheath. The term *tenosynovitis* is commonly applied to those conditions at the wrist (colloquially labelled 'teno' in the workplace) that are characterized by discomfort, tenderness and pain on stretching. Histologically, features more akin to tendon degeneration rather than inflammation are found (Figure 5.6), and purists prefer the term 'tenovaginitis' for conditions such as de Quervain's disease.

Tenovaginitis stenosans accurately describes the condition of trigger thumb or trigger finger, in which the fibrous sheath tightens around the flexor tendon.

It is conceded elsewhere in this text that it is reprehensible for the label 'teno' to be applied indiscriminately by medical practitioners, usually family practitioners who have first contact with patients, to pain in the wrist – which may have many causes. Incorrect labelling may lead to unwanted consequences, particularly the adoption of the role of claimant/litigant by a patient.

However, tenosynovitis is *common*; indeed it is far better that the possibility of the existence of this condition is explored, and appropriate measures undertaken if necessary, than tenosynovitis be allowed to develop into its chronic form. Medical practitioners should advise their patients that the development of a work-related upper limb disorder does not necessarily infer negligence or liability for damages on the part of the employer. It is true that the diagnosis of a work-related disorder by the attending doctor may engender a sense of aggrievement in the patient, particularly if the work environment is stressful; however, in my opinion, there is a greater risk of aggrievement when medical specialists fail to appreciate the subtleties of diagnosis and deny genuine patients appropriate advice and management strategies in the less than florid case.

In this text, tenosynovitis is used synonymously with tenovaginitis.

Pathophysiology

Tendons are subject to tensile, compression and shear forces. Plasticity (deformation of collagen fibrils with subsequent reformation) is a normal feature of physiological collagenous activity. If the rate of microstructural catabolism as a consequence of uncompensatable deformation is greater than anabolic reconstitution some degree of *functional failure* occurs.

Histologically, the biopsy findings in conditions such as de Quervain's tenovaginitis are less characteristic of inflammation (in which one would expect an invasion of inflammatory cells) than degeneration. There is increased fibroblastic activity and vascular proliferation but, particularly, an increase in glycosaminoglycan content (hyaluronic acid, chondroitin sulphate and dermatan sulphate). Synovial thickening and fibrocartilaginous transformation are usually found. The changes in collagen fibre size and orientation and the overall reduced collagen content, increased deposition of proteoglycan between the fibres, and increase in cell numbers in shoulder tendon lesions are stated to be consistent with inflammation and a fibro-proliferative response to trauma such as impingement and hypoxia (Cawston *et al.*, 1996).

Epistemological errors result from the contrived 'need' for the detection of inflammatory changes in order to make a specific diagnosis of activity-related tenosynovitis. **Overuse leads to degradative changes (tendinosis).** These should be interpreted as the *response to stress* and not merely the inevitable ('constitutional') age-related changes of degeneration.

In addition to overuse, other aetiological factors, such as metabolic, hormonal and anatomical, may need to be considered. Shear forces may be relevant in some cases, for instance in de Quervain's disease in which tendons angulate sharply over bony surfaces. Rheumatoid arthritis should always be considered, particularly when there are more florid manifestations of inflammatory synovitis (such as in some cases of extensor tenosynovitis).

It is worth stressing that it is disingenuous to view the degenerative changes of tendinosis as simply age-related, uninfluenced by activity, and therefore 'constitutional': these morphological changes become symptomatic as a result of overload. From the legal standpoint, occupational, domestic, recreational, or sports-related factors may be causative or aggravating.

De Quervain's disease

Tillaux in 1892 described this condition that he labelled 'tenosynovitis crépitante or d'ai'. Fritz de Quervain labelled the condition that now bears his name 'fibrose, stenosierende tendovaginitis' in 1895. It is a discrete condition, affecting the tendons of extensor pollicis brevis (EPB) and abductor pollicis longus (APL). The site of the lesion is the *first dorsal compartment* of the wrist at the level of the radial styloid (Figure 5.7). The extensor retinaculum retains the tendons in their fibro-osseous canal at this anatomical site.

Workers at risk are those engaged in activities requiring repetitive use of the thumb, as in the pinch grip, and repetitive radio-ulnar deviations at the wrist. Leao (1958) stated that de Quervain's disease could be considered an occupational disease in many cases: in his

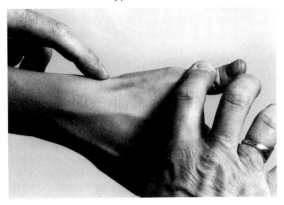

Figure 5.7 The tendons of extensor pollicis brevis (EPB) and abductor pollicis longus (APL) are demonstrated on resisted contraction of thumb extension

series there was a high percentage of domestic workers. Mothers of young children are another at-risk group (Harvey *et al.*, 1990).

Activity-related discomfort is experienced over the radial aspect of the wrist and forearm. In the acute phase crepitus is sometimes experienced, but it is an inconstant feature. Patients are usually aware of swelling of the distal forearm.

The pain may radiate proximally and distally. It is related to manual activities, particularly those requiring frequent deviations of the wrist in the transverse plane. Initially, the symptoms lessen overnight and at weekends. Progressively, they intrude to a greater extent at work and, eventually, discomfort is experienced during all manual activities at home as well as at work.

The positive physical signs are those to be expected of a lesion affecting a contractile structure: pain on resisted contraction and on stretching. Resisted extension and resisted abduction of the thumb are painful in the acute phase. The most reliable sign is pain on stretching the affected tendons. Finkelstein's test is the application of passive ulnar deviation at the wrist combined with passive flexion of the thumb across the palm (see Figure 7.28). The examiner should apply pressure to the radial margin of the second metacarpal to procure ulnar deviation at the wrist. When positive, pain is reproduced over the radial styloid. Tenderness is localized to the affected tendons; it may be found at the radial aspect of the radial styloid or just distally overlying

the radiocarpal joint. Often there is swelling over the radial styloid (Figure 5.7).

In the chronic case, in which fibrotic stenosis of the tendon sheaths occurs, the application of Finkelstein's test reveals loss of range of thumb flexion across the palm. Localized tenderness is a constant feature prior to full resolution of the condition.

Management strategies include the use of non-steroidal anti-inflammatory drugs, anti-inflammatory physiotherapeutic modalities, wrist/thumb spica splintage, steroid injections and surgery. Initially, a period of reduced strain upon the affected limb may be combined with NSAIDs. However, anti-inflammatory management by ice and ultrasound/laser or by NSAIDs is often disappointing in efficacy. Steroid injections, when performed with expertise, offer a more rapid response, but they should still be combined with an appropriate period of respite from provocative stress.

Wrist immobilization is usually unnecessary; when used it should include a thumb spica to abolish all activity of the affected tendons. In general, the use of immobilization of joints for protection of the soft tissues is to be eschewed. Degradation of the articular surfaces of the immobilized joints may occur. Loss of muscle tone in adjacent muscle groups is disadvantageous as rehabilitation may then be prolonged.

Steroid infiltration should be performed by injecting around and along the line of the affected tendons at the level of the radial styloid or just proximal to the base of the first metacarpal (Figure 5.8). An appropriate dosage is 10 mg of triamcinolone. It may be mixed with 1 ml of 1% lignocaine in a 2 ml syringe; a 23 gauge needle is ideal. Harvey *et al.* (1990) reported 80% resolution of de Quervain's disease with steroid injections; accuracy of injection was stressed. In my experience, more than one injection may be necessary for the condition to resolve completely. A review at 3 weeks after the initial injection should be made and a further injection given if necessary.

Surgical decompression is advocated by some authors but is usually unnecessary unless the chronic form is encountered in which there is marked fibrotic stenosis of the first dorsal compartment.

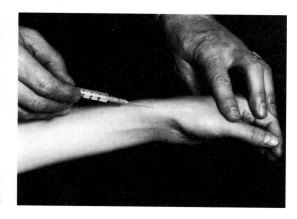

Figure 5.8 Injection of the tendon sheaths of EPB and APL is demonstrated

De Quervain's disease must be differentiated from osteoarthritis of the first carpometacarpal (CMC) joint (see Figure 7.32). In the latter condition tenderness is more anterior, and passive abduction and extension of the first metacarpal at the CMC joint are painful. A confirmatory test is exacerbation of symptoms on axial compression combined with rotation of the thumb metacarpal (the grind test). Axial loading of the thumb combined with passive flexion and extension of the metacarpal constitutes the crank test (Pellegrini, 1992). Differentiation from intersection syndrome is made by the exact localization of tenderness and swelling. Very occasionally, a burning type of discomfort may be felt over the distal radial styloid in cases of superficial radial nerve entrapment (Wartenberg's syndrome).

Intersection syndrome

Pain, crepitus and swelling are the cardinal features of this condition, which arises at the locus in the forearm at which the tendons of EPB and APL cross over the radial extensors – the ECRL and ECRB (Figure 5.9). It is otherwise known as peritendinitis crepitans, reflecting the inflammatory reaction of the paratenon at the level of the musculotendinous junction of the affected thumb tendons.

It is probably very common. It is difficult to estimate its true incidence, however, as it is rarely distinguished, either clinically or in annotation, from de Quervain's tenosynovitis by medical practitioners in family practice.

In their oft-quoted monograph on its industrial causation, Thompson *et al.* (1951) cited Velpeau as the first to describe the condition; it was labelled 'cellulite peritendineuse' in his textbook published in 1841. Troell (1918) used the term tendovaginitis crepitans, comparing it to a similar condition affecting the tendons of the lower leg, including the Achilles tendon.

It is undoubtedly an overuse phenomenon. Numerous pathophysiological theories have been propounded to explain its crepitating nature. These include a myotendinosis of APL and EPB, the development of an adventitious bursa between the contents of the two compartments, and a tenosynovitis of the underlying radial wrist extensors (ECRL and ECRB). Thompson considered that unaccustomed work or a return to work after a period of absence were the stressors in a significant proportion of cases. Patients' complaints include pain, swelling, tenderness, creaking (crepitus) and a feeling of weakness. A sticky fibrinous deposit between the tendons of the first and second dorsal compartment is often found in those cases subjected to surgery.

In sport, rowers and canoeists are frequently affected; weight-lifters and dog handlers are other vulnerable groups (Hutson, 1996). In the workplace, manual workers in industry constitute the highest risk group, but it also occurs in other groups such as agricultural workers. In Thompson's series in 544 patients with forearm tendinitis, 419 cases were due to peritendinitis crepitans. Most of these occurred in the Vauxhall motor factory.

Intersection syndrome may be differentiated from de Quervain's disease by virtue of its site – some 4–8 cm proximal to Lister's tubercle. Crepitus is a constant feature in the acute state; it is both audible and palpable. Finkelstein's test may be positive. Tenderness is usually marked, and it is the last sign to disappear prior to complete resolution. Localized, fusiform swelling is present, particularly in the acute stage.

Infiltration of steroid and local anaesthetic is the preferred treatment. The symptoms and signs resolve so quickly (within a few days) that other management strategies, for instance immobilization or ultrasound and transverse friction massage, are very much second best. As with other tendinopathies, an appraisal of the causative and/or provocative factors

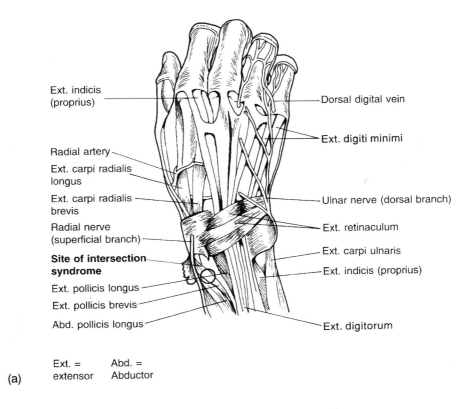

Ext. indicis (proprius)

Dorsal digital vein

Ext. digiti minimi

Radial artery

Ext. carpi radialis longus

Ext. carpi radialis brevis

Radial nerve (superficial branch)

Site of intersection syndrome

Ext. pollicis longus

Ext. pollicis brevis

Abd. pollicis longus

Ulnar nerve (dorsal branch)

Ext. retinaculum

Ext. carpi ulnaris

Ext. indicis (proprius)

Ext. digitorum

Ext. = extensor   Abd. = Abductor

(a)

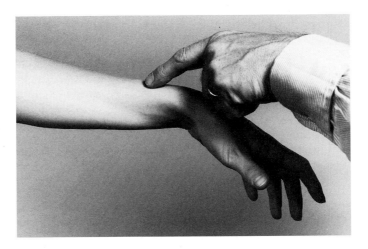

(b)

Figure 5.9 Intersection syndrome occurs at the crossover between the tendons of extensor pollicis brevis/abductor pollicis longus and the extensores carpi radialis: (*a*) illustrated diagrammatically; (*b*) demonstrated clinically

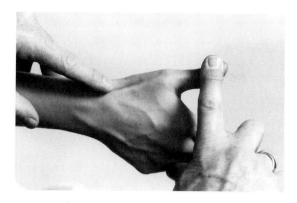

Figure 5.10 Extensor pollicis longus is demonstrated

should be made. Work schedules usually need to be modified to allow complete resolution of the condition. A state of increased vulnerability to recurrence of symptoms persists for months and possibly for some years thereafter.

Extensor pollicis longus tendinitis

Other than as a component of rheumatoid arthritis, tendinitis of extensor pollicis longus (EPL) – the constituent of the *third dorsal compartment* – is relatively uncommon (Figures 5.10, 5.11). As an overuse syndrome, tendinitis (or even rupture, as in 'drummer boy palsy' – an injury first reported in Prussian drummers by Dums in 1896) arises as a result of attrition at Lister's tubercle. This may also be caused by a fracture of the radial styloid, as in a minimally displaced Colles' fracture.

The clinical findings of tendinitis are pain on passive flexion and loss of full passive flexion of the thumb, localized tenderness and swelling at Lister's tubercle, and pain on resisted thumb extension. When attrition leads to rupture of the EPL, there is gross weakness of active extension of the distal phalanx of the thumb.

Extensor indicis proprius syndrome

A stenosing tenovaginitis of the extensor indicis proprius tendon is said to occur as a result of excessive activity of the finger extensors. Pain on attempted extension of the index finger against resistance from a position of full wrist flexion is stated to be an essential clinical

finding (Spinner and Olshansky, 1973). Tenderness is localized to the affected area on the dorsum of the wrist, approximately 1 cm to the ulnar side of Lister's tubercle (Figure 5.11). Management strategies are identical to those for the tendinopathies affecting the first to the third dorsal components.

Extensor digitorum tenosynovitis

This condition of the *fourth dorsal compartment* may assume a florid form as part of rheumatoid arthritis. It is rarely caused by overuse. Swelling distal to the extensor retinaculum may be marked, sometimes in the shape of a goose foot (Figure 5.12). When due to rheumatoid arthritis it is commonly an isolated lesion in the hand. Dysfunction of the hand is often little affected unless rupture of one or more tendons occurs with a chronic lesion.

Extensor digiti minimi tendinitis

Stenosing tenovaginitis of the *fifth dorsal compartment* has been reported after trauma and after overuse, but it is rare (Hooper and McMaster, 1979). In the case described by Hooper, which may have been associated with an extreme amount of handwriting, there were clinical and histopathological similarities to de Quervain's disease. Tenderness was detected immediately distal to the head of the ulna. Attempting to flex the wrist after making a fist provoked pain.

Extensor carpi ulnaris tendinitis

Tendinitis of extensor carpi ulnaris (ECU) within the *sixth dorsal compartment* is probably the next most common extensor tendinitis after the tendinopathies affecting the first and second dorsal compartments. Groups at risk are those in whom radio-ulnar wrist deviations and forearm rotations are frequent, for instance machinists and professional golfers.

Provocative tests include passive radial deviation of the wrist with a fully pronated forearm; attempts by the patient to procure the same movement are equally painful (see Figure 7.27). Surprisingly, perhaps, full passive supination also provokes discomfort. Resisted dorsiflexion of the wrist and resisted ulnar deviation of the wrist are painful in the acute phase. Tenderness is detected over the

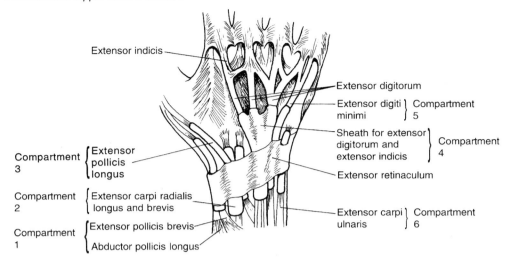

Extensor indicis

Extensor digitorum

Extensor digiti } Compartment
minimi   5

Sheath for extensor } Compartment
digitorum and   4
extensor indicis

Extensor retinaculum

Compartment { Extensor
3   pollicis
            longus

Compartment { Extensor carpi radialis
2   longus and brevis

Compartment { Extensor pollicis brevis
1   Abductor pollicis longus

Extensor carpi } Compartment
ulnaris   6

(a)

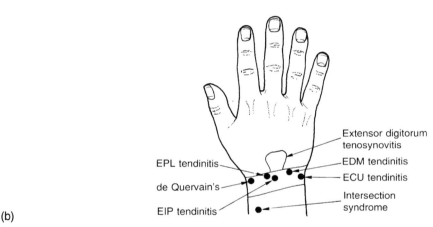

Extensor digitorum
tenosynovitis

EPL tendinitis

de Quervain's

EIP tendinitis

EDM tendinitis

ECU tendinitis

Intersection
syndrome

(b)

Figure 5.11 (*a*) The dorsal compartments of the wrist are illustrated; (*b*) the sites of tenderness are indicated

ulnar styloid, along the centimetre or so of the ulna proximal to the styloid process, and along the line of the tendon immediately distal to the styloid process.

Occasionally, subluxation of the ECU is a causative factor. This may be brought about by active supination of the ulnar-deviated wrist. Clicking is a frequent complaint.

In the most frequent, less florid, case the provocation of pain on passive radial deviation of the wrist with full pronation of the forearm is the most constant feature. ECU tendinitis should be differentiated from a lesion of the inferior radio-ulnar joint, from a ganglion that may be found occasionally to the ulnar side of the wrist, and from a sprain of the ulnar collateral ligament of the wrist. In these conditions there is no pain on resisted muscle contraction. Precise palpation has considerable discriminant value.

Flexor carpi ulnaris tendinitis

Flexor carpi ulnaris (FCU) tendinitis is probably the most commonly diagnosed flexor tendinitis. Even so, it is much less common than

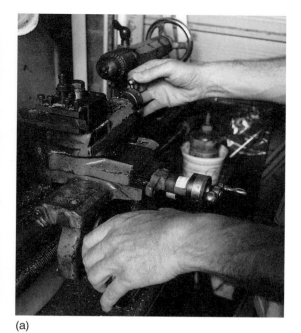

(a)

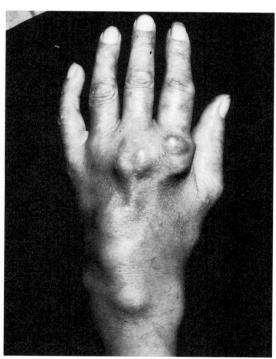

(b)

Figure 5.12 (*a*) This extensor tenosynovitis was an isolated lesion on the dorsum of the left hand of a lathe operator. (*b*) Extensor digitorum tenosynovitis is often due to rheumatoid arthritis. An established condition is illustrated

the extensor tendinopathies. (NB: see below, Flexor digitorum tendinitis.)

It may be difficult to decide whether FCU tendinitis results from repetitive direct trauma to the region of the pisiform bone or from repetitive flexion movements of the wrist.

In racquet players, or those sportsmen who grasp a bat or club, direct transmission of forces may give rise to a fracture of the pisiform (or hamate), piso-triquetral chondromalacia ('sesamoiditis'), or flexor carpi ulnaris tendinitis. Industrial workers or those employed in the building/demolition industries are also at risk of developing these conditions from heavy hammer work.

Pain, tenderness and swelling are usually localized to the affected tendon, just proximal to the pisiform. Resisted wrist flexion and resisted ulnar deviation of the wrist are painful. Passive stretching of the FCU tendon by combined extension and radial deviation of the wrist provokes discomfort. Pisiform pathologies are characterized by pain on compressing the pisiform against the underlying triquetral bone.

Calcific tendinitis, a dystrophic condition, is occasionally seen. Its features are similar to calcific tendinitis occurring elsewhere (for instance in the supraspinatus tendon). It gives rise to pain of acute onset and exquisite tenderness. Additionally, swelling and erythema are present (which may give rise to the mistaken impression that the condition is infective – whereas it is actually inflammatory/degenerative). Unaccustomed use of the hand may be a triggering activity.

FCU tendinitis may be associated with entrapment neuropathy of the deep branch of the ulnar nerve in Guyon's canal, during its course around the pisiform. More usually, however, compression neuropathy arises independently, for instance in those workers who use pliers or screwdrivers repetitively or in sport, as in handlebar neuropathy of cyclists.

A suitable management strategy for FCU tendinitis is the combination of active intervention in the form of steroid/local anaesthetic injection and relative or absolute rest depending upon its severity. Measures should be undertaken to reduce direct trauma to, or compression of, the pisiform region of the wrist, and to reduce the frequency of repeated wrist flexion and/or ulnar deviation.

Flexor carpi radialis tendinitis

Although referred to and researched by Thorson and Szabo (1992), flexor carpi radialis tendinitis appears to be relatively uncommon. In my own practice a patient presenting with acute calcific tendinitis experienced severe pain on attempted use of the hand (Figure 5.13). Pain is felt in the volar radial aspect of the wrist at the base of the thenar eminence. The diagnosis is based on the provocation of pain on resisted palmarflexion of the wrist, and pain on resisted radial deviation of the wrist.

Flexor digitorum tendinitis

This is usually seen in association with median nerve entrapment neuropathy in the carpal tunnel (the carpal tunnel syndrome – CTS). Although the association between flexor tendinitis and carpal tunnel syndrome is denied by some observers, a careful clinical examination may reveal otherwise. Undoubtedly, flexor tendinitis may have a causal relationship with manual activities in industrial workers, and may give rise to median nerve compression. With appropriate early management, progression of tendinitis or CTS may be aborted. This 'transient' case may not reach the portals of the hospital specialist and its true incidence is probably unrecognized.

Sometimes, a more chronic stenosing form of flexor tenosynovitis (tenovaginitis) arises, and this is usually associated with a refractory form of carpal tunnel syndrome. However, the two conditions (flexor tendinitis and CTS) should be distinguishable clinically.

Flexor digitorum tendinitis is characterized by discomfort on passive extension of the fingers, particularly with a dorsiflexed wrist. In the relatively acute phase swelling may be observed immediately proximal to the wrist creases (Kiefhaber and Stern, 1992). If the condition is allowed to become chronic, fixed flexion contractures of the digits occur. Patients comment on their inability to straighten their fingers fully, and on discomfort associated with attempts to do so. Power of finger flexion is usually well maintained,

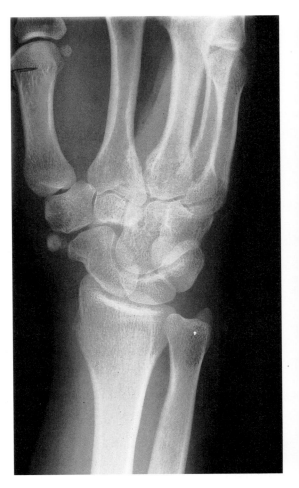

Figure 5.13 Calcification is demonstrated in the flexor carpi radialis tendon on this radiograph. (From Hutson, M.A., 1996, by permission)

though isometric contraction may be accompanied by discomfort. The 'reversed Phalen's sign' is positive: an attempt by the patient to maintain dorsiflexion of the opposed wrists with extended fingers provokes discomfort (see Figure 7.26b). (Compare Phalen's sign when median nerve entrapment symptoms are provoked in cases of CTS.) Naturally, if CTS is caused by chronic flexor tendinitis in an individual patient, a positive Phalen's test and a positive reversed Phalen's test may coexist.

Workers engaged in tasks requiring repetitive grasping, and the use of a strong grip, particularly assembly line workers, are at risk. In my experience, the group of young patients described by Szabo and Madison (1992) as developing CTS during the course of repetitive manual labour are likely to have an underlying flexor tendinitis. They would be expected to recover fully with rest.

CTS is described fully in the subsection on Entrapment neuropathies, below.

Stenosing tenovaginitis of the digital flexors (trigger finger; trigger thumb)

The essential feature of this condition is thickening of the first annular (A1) pulley of the fibrous flexor tendon sheath at the level of the metacarpophalangeal (MCP) joints. This gives a triggering effect during flexion and extension. The lesion is palpable as a tender nodule overlying the volar aspect of the MCP joint. Clicking as well as triggering is often noticed by the patient. It usually affects the thumb, middle or ring fingers.

Its causation is open to dispute inasmuch as a vulnerability to soft tissue lesions of this type may exist in a subgroup of the general population – a low-grade 'rheumatological' diathesis, but without the overt manifestations of arthritis. Numerous activities on assembly lines demand strong grasping of objects of a sufficient size to occupy most of the palm. It seems logical, if unproven, that repetitive direct pressure upon the distal palm crease in combination with digital flexor contractions during grasping is the causative activity. Some studies have demonstrated an increased incidence in the dominant hand. Bonnici and Spencer (1988) found an increased incidence in females and an association with occupations that involve repetitive hand movements. Sporting activities are a further cause of trigger finger.

The treatment of choice is injection of steroid within the tendon sheath: 5 mg triamcinolone is sufficient, using a 23 gauge needle. Some authors advance the tip of the needle through the tendon to the bone behind, then withdraw slightly before injecting to ensure reaching the retrotendon space (and thereby avoiding injecting into the tendon). I find this is unnecessary: with the use of a needle bent to 30 degrees within its guard, the injection may be made parallel to the tendon within the sheath.

Early relief of discomfort and triggering is the expected outcome following injection. Marks and Gunther (1989), Rhoades *et al.* (1984) and Quinnell (1980) reported high success rates with injection treatments. Lapidus and Guidotti (1972) changed their management strategy for cases of de Quervain's disease and stenosing tenovaginitis of the digits from surgery to local injection of steroids with considerable success. Refractory cases usually respond satisfactorily to surgical release.

GANGLION (SYNOVIAL CYST)

A ganglion is a tense cystic swelling that is associated with a joint or tendon sheath. It comprises a fibrous sheath surrounding a synovial membrane, and enclosing thick viscous fluid. A common site is the dorsum of the wrist, where there is tethering to the carpal joints or extensor tendons. Ganglions are also seen on the volar aspect of the wrist (Figure 5.14), around the ankle and foot, and occasionally elsewhere. They are found most frequently at between 20 and 30 years of age, with a female : male predominance of 2 : 1 (Nelson *et al.*, 1972).

A ganglion is often painless, but may become painful for no obvious reason and then interfere with normal function of the wrist. Its aetiology is obscure; accordingly, its association with occupations that demand repetitive wrist flexion and extension must be presumptive in individual cases. It is not a manifestation of a rheumatic diathesis and should easily be differentiated from the synovial proliferation of rheumatoid arthritis. Occasionally, when patients complain of activity-related dorsal wrist pain but there is no evidence of swelling and no signs of tendinitis, an occult dorsal wrist ganglion may be suspected.

There are usually no features of tendinitis on examination. Firm pressure over the ganglion is painful, and the wrist movements may be minimally restricted. In the event of pain during everyday activities the ganglion may be punctured using a 20 gauge needle. (Nothing less will do.) Alternatively, dispersal of the viscous fluid may be achieved by firm manual pressure, or the traditional use of a heavy object such as a Victorian family Bible. Recurrence is relatively common, in which case excision may be performed. As the surgeon may be faced with a tedious dissection,

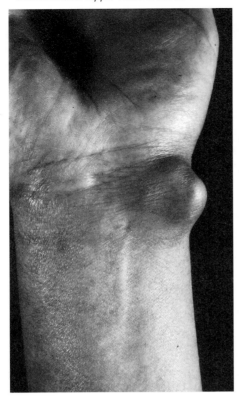

Figure 5.14 Although ganglions are usually found on the dorsum of the wrist, they may occur elsewhere. When present on the volar aspect of the wrist, as in this case, they are particularly subject to recurrence after surgical excision

surgery should only be contemplated when the symptoms are intrusive.

In Nelson's series of 222 patients (in whom 57% of ganglions occurred over the dorsal aspect of the wrist) the cure rate of a group treated by digital pressure (66%) compared favourably with a group treated by aspiration and triamcinolone injection (65%). However the most successful treatment was surgical: an 84% cure rate with surgery under local anaesthetic and 94% cure rate with surgery under general anaesthesia.

DUPUYTREN'S CONTRACTURE

This condition, comprising a progressive thickening and contracture of the palmar fascia, was first described by Baron Dupuytren in 1834. He observed the condition in a coachman and in a wine merchant, and considered that repetitive manual activities were causative.

Dupuytren's contracture often affects the plantar fascia too in those who have lesions in the hands. It is more common in men than women, and is uncommon under the age of 40 years. The rate of progression is variable, but worsening contracture is inexorable.

The palmar fascia is intimately associated with the overlying skin. The earliest sign of the condition is nodular thickening of the palmar fascia in the palm. The skin soon becomes hypertrophic and puckered, however, and the affected finger or fingers develop a flexion deformity (Figure 5.15). The ring finger is almost always affected, the little and middle fingers less severely in the early stages.

The aetiology is unclear and is undoubtedly multifactorial (Noble *et al.*, 1992). It is more

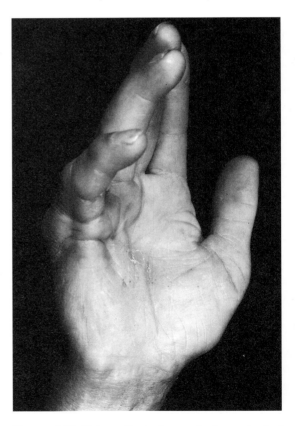

Figure 5.15 This patient demonstrates a typical Dupuytren's contracture. The ring and little fingers are predominantly affected

common in Europe than in the USA, and is rarely seen in non-Caucasians. It often has a familial distribution. There is an increased incidence in epileptics and in chronic alcoholics. It is postulated that frequent firm grasping may be the aetiological factor in some patients. However, the common association with contracture of the plantar fascia indicates that constitutional factors are paramount. Surgical excision of the affected tissue is the only method of reducing the tendency to severe flexion contracture, but recurrence occurs in a significant proportion of patients.

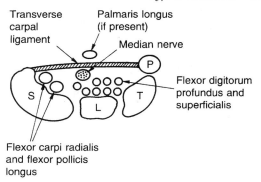

Figure 5.16 The carpal tunnel at the level of the proximal row of carpal bones

ENTRAPMENT NEUROPATHIES

Acute compression or chronic irritation/compression of the median, ulnar and radial nerves and their branches may occur at the elbow, in the forearm or in the hand. Injuries in the former group include acute compression neuropathies secondary to fracture (not considered in this text) or to contusion of the adjacent soft tissues in the workplace. Most chronic entrapment neuropathies have several contributory factors, including adverse mechanics (for instance, reduced capacity of the carpal tunnel or tight fascial tunnels around the elbow), overuse or overload, and (possibly) the double crush phenomenon in which increased susceptibility is caused by mild cervical radiculopathy.

Pathological changes include focal demyelination, giving rise to a neuropraxia and conduction block in the early case, and Wallerian (distal) degeneration in the advanced case. When sufficiently severe, the neural compression is revealed by electrodiagnostic tests; typical abnormalities include prolonged distal latency and slowing of nerve conduction velocity across a specific segment.

The clinical features include pain, paraesthesia and numbness, weakness, muscle atrophy and varying degrees of sensory loss. However, a high index of suspicion is required to differentiate from more proximal lesions, such as cervical radiculopathy or thoracic outlet syndrome. In this regard it should be noted that peripheral nerve entrapment may give rise to proximal discomfort and,

peripherally, to vague, episodic and 'non-classical' symptoms.

The median nerve

Carpal tunnel syndrome

At the wrist the median nerve is a mixed nerve, supplying the muscles of thumb opposition (opponens pollicis, abductor pollicis brevis and flexor pollicis brevis) and the lateral two lumbricals, and sensation to the radial three and a half digits. The carpal tunnel, through which it passes with the finger flexor tendons, is a fibro-osseous channel, bounded by the carpal bones and the transverse carpal ligament (Figures 5.16, 5.17).

Carpal tunnel syndrome (CTS) is produced by entrapment of the median nerve in the carpal tunnel. It is probably the most commonly encountered peripheral entrapment neuropathy and has been the subject of much debate, particularly with respect to its compensatability.

Historically, it was not until the report in *The Lancet* by Brain, Wright and Wilkinson (1947) that CTS was recognized to be a compression neuropathy of the median nerve in the carpal tunnel. Prior to that, although the sensory manifestations and the motor findings had been recognized since the previous century, most patients were diagnosed as having a lesion of the brachial plexus (in the case of those with dominant sensory symptoms) or a compression of the thenar motor branch of the median nerve (in patients with thenar atrophy and weakness). Brain (subsequently

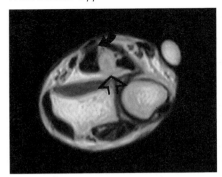

(a)

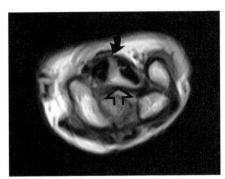

(b)

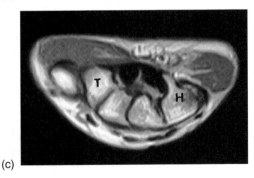

(c)

Figure 5.17 A space-occupying lesion such as a ganglion (illustrated on this MRI scan) may cause compression of the median nerve in the carpal tunnel. Sequence of post-gadolinium enhancing images: (*a*) proximal to the carpal tunnel, the marker is on the ulnar side: a ganglion (*open arrow*) appears as a rim enhancing mass separating the flexor tendons, where the median nerve (*curved arrow*) is more superficial but deep to the palmaris longus tendon;
(*b*) At the level of the scaphoid and the pisiform, the flexor retinaculum is bowed with the median nerve compressed by the deeper enhancing ganglion;
(*c*) at the level of the trapezium (**T**) and the hook of hamate (**H**) the distal extent of the ganglion is demonstrated with the flexor tendons less separated. (Courtesy of J.K. Fairbairn, Lister Bestcare MRI Unit, Nottingham City Hospital)

Lord Brain) and his colleagues considered that ischaemia of the median nerve resulted from repetitive *extensions* of the wrist.

Subsequently, in 1950, Phalen wrote the first of his articles on CTS, which was by then recognized as an entrapment neuropathy that was usually non-traumatic in origin and unassociated with other medical conditions. An interesting account by Pfeffer *et al.* of the history of carpal tunnel syndrome was published in the *Journal of Hand Surgery* in 1988.

Epidemiology and aetiology

There is an association with pregnancy, rheumatoid arthritis, myxoedema and diabetes, and also with space-occupying lesions (including swollen flexor tendon synovia) within the carpal tunnel. Phalen (1966, 1972) wrote authoritatively of the carpal tunnel syndrome and concluded that thickening of the flexor synovialis in CTS 'must be associated with some type of rheumatic process in the great majority of patients'. He defended his view by stating that the improvement after localized steroid injections was consistent with a rheumatic origin; additionally, he observed a frequent association with other 'rheumatic' diseases such as trigger finger, de Quervain's disease, tennis elbow and periarthritis of the shoulder.

In the context of present-day knowledge and debate, Phalen's arguments become somewhat circular, being dependent upon the concept that the aforementioned conditions are 'rheumatic' in the strict inflammatory sense – now disputed, of course. He noted that 'thickening of the flexor synovialis may be caused by prolonged forceful grasping movements . . . under these (exceedingly rare) conditions carpal tunnel syndrome could be classified as an industrial disease'. He noted a 3 : 1 female to male ratio and an incidence of 78% between 40 and 70 years of age.

Szabo and Madison (1992) have commented upon a second, distinct, population of CTS patients, a younger group of workers of both sexes who experience symptoms at work. Braun *et al.* (1989) labelled work-related symptoms that resolved with rest, elevation or conservative treatment as **dynamic** carpal tunnel syndrome. They confirmed the diagnosis of (D)CTS by volumetric tests, provocative stress tests (which involved simulated work conditions) and sensory testing.

Affected patients had sensory impairment and significant swelling after provocative stress.

Masear *et al.* (1986) noted a high incidence of CTS, sufficiently severe to require surgery, in a group of workers in a meat packing plant undertaking (boning) activities that required repetitive movements of the wrists. The comparison was made with workers doing jobs with less repetitive manual activity such as those on the loading deck, and with the general population. Amongst other researchers, Wieslander *et al.* (1989) have identified an association with repetitive tasks that involve flexion and extension of the wrist, strong grip, or exposure to vibration. *Inter alia*, meat packers, supermarket check-out clerks and assembly line workers are at risk.

Feldman *et al.* (1987) refer to an increased incidence in cashiers, card sorters, hairdressers, small part assemblers (including electronic assembly workers), garment stitchers and butchers. In particular, they studied the incidence of CTS in workers having what they termed high-risk and low-risk jobs in an electronics assembly plant. Workers on the high-risk jobs, such as welding and integrated line work which required repetitive 'exertional flexion–extension–pinching motions', were more likely than those in low-risk jobs to suffer from hand symptoms suggestive of CTS, a positive Phalen's test, or hand weakness.

Silverstein *et al.* (1987) used videotapes and electromyographic (EMG) studies to estimate hand force and repetitiveness when assessing 574 workers from six industries. Significant positive associations were observed between 'hand wrist CTDs' (cumulative trauma disorders, which included carpal tunnel syndrome) and high force–high repetition jobs. The authors considered that the negative association between hand wrist CTDs and age and years on the job suggested survival bias.

Smith *et al.* (1977) produced experimental data from cadaver hands to support the hypothesis that the median nerve is subjected to compression against the flexor retinaculum by tensed overlying flexor tendons. They concluded that repetitive hand activities involving pinch or grasp *during wrist flexion* may be a contributing factor in some cases of CTS.

Cyriax (1969) considered that repeated use of the hand extended at the wrist compresses the median nerve against the carpal bones. In this respect he came to the same conclusion as Lord Brain. Cyriax stated that scrubbing on hands and knees, or using clippers, were aetiological factors.

Occupational exposure to vibration may cause carpal tunnel syndrome (Rosenbaum and Ochoa, 1993). Lundborg *et al.* (1987) has noted an association between CTS in male patients and exposure to hand-held vibrating tools. Symptoms and electrodiagnostic abnormalities consistent with CTS were found by Koskimies *et al.* (1990) in 20% of forestry workers who were exposed to the vibration of chain saws.

Nathan *et al.* (1988) conducted a cross-sectional study among a general population of working adults. They were 'unable to establish any consistent association between the occurrence of impaired nerve conduction of the median nerve and occupational class or the level of hand activity'.

The atypicality of clinical presentation in many patients has led to a further theory to account for the vulnerability of the median nerve. The concept of the 'double crush syndrome' was described by Upton and McComas in 1973, and clearly has its advocates. In 115 patients with electrodiagnostic evidence of an entrapment neuropathy, involving the median nerve or the ulnar nerve or both, there was evidence of a 'cervical root' lesion in 81 (70%). The 'evidence' for the root lesion came from several sources, including the radiological demonstration of cervical spondylosis, complaints of neck pain and stiffness, and a previous history of neck injury in many subjects as well as clinical and EMG evidence of a root syndrome. The essence of the hypothesis is 'that neural function is impaired because single axons, having been compressed in one region, become especially susceptible to damage at another site'.

Medicolegal aspects
In their recent erudite and wide-ranging review of median nerve disorders, Rosenbaum and Ochoa (1993) state that there is

widespread recognition of the relationship between hand and wrist use and symptoms of carpal tunnel syndrome . . . a correlation between manual activity and detection of cases of carpal tunnel syndrome has been shown most convincingly in meat and poultry processors, electronics assemblers, garment workers, aircraft workers, and frozen food processors.

In a reasoned approach to the subject, they identify the need for an established dose–response relation and a temporal relation between reputed cause and effect, as well as biological plausibility and statistical correlation, to support the causal nature of the association. It is generally recognized that some statistical data should be interpreted with caution, yet the nihilistic approach of some authors, such as Hadler (1993), to suggestions for a causal role for occupation should be eschewed.

As compensation depends upon an informed and well-reasoned medical opinion, diagnosis must be established and a causal relationship (if it exists) identified. Non-occupational activities and underlying conditions may be relevant. It is apparent to all observers that symptoms from a pre-existing carpal tunnel syndrome may indeed be aggravated by work activities; it is also accepted that symptoms from CTS (from other causes) may arise in workers. Dose–response and temporal relationships need to be established in individual cases to support a causal association between work and the development of the condition.

When associated with the use of hand-held vibrating tools, carpal tunnel syndrome is a prescribed disease (PD A12) in the UK. The Regulations appertaining to the Prescribed Occupational Diseases (Social Security Regulations 1975) have been reviewed relatively recently but no changes have been made. In their report on work-related upper limb disorders (and whether they should be prescribed) presented to the UK Secretary of State for Social Security in 1992, the Industrial Injuries Advisory Council stated that little weight should be given to surveys in which there were no data on controls without the condition. The Council noted the apparent high rates of CTS in selected groups, but 'the findings are difficult to interpret'. They concluded that the epidemiological evidence for the association between CTS and the use of hand-held vibrating tools was sufficiently strong for it to be compensatable: '*Exceptionally* [my italics], carpal tunnel syndrome should be prescribed

in such a way that individual cases are considered for compensation.'

Pathoanatomy/pathophysiology

As the causes of CTS include space-occupying lesions, pathological conditions such as benign tumours, ganglions (see Figure 5.17), amyloidosis, chondrocalcinosis and florid (rheumatological) flexor tenosynovitis may be revealed if suspected on scanning or at surgery.

In general, when patients with CTS are submitted to biopsy at the time of surgery, thickening of the synovial lining of the flexor tendons is a constant histological feature (Figure 5.18). In the majority of cases the changes are not typical of inflammation. (Nevertheless, the clinical association of some cases of CTS with flexor tenovaginitis/tenosynovitis strongly suggests that repetitive flexion and extension of the wrist are the most common related activities.)

Braun *et al.* (1989) have suggested that reversible ischaemic impairment of the median nerve is the pathophysiological mechanism in the younger patient group involved in manual labour. Their explanation for 'dynamic' carpal tunnel syndrome is that the condition is influenced by wrist dynamics and fluid pressures. In chronic CTS, nerve conduction studies are usually abnormal; morphological damage to the median nerve then becomes permanent.

The distinction between the early and late cases has a practical bearing. The early 'dynamic' case will respond to intracarpal tunnel steroid injections followed by the avoidance of provocative activities. The late case is irreversible to the extent that it is unlikely to resolve spontaneously or with conservative treatment; surgical intervention is then indicated. The diagnosis should never be delayed until signs of motor dysfunction (which are usually permanent) are apparent.

Clinical features

The typical patient suffers from pain and paraesthesia in the distribution of the median nerve: the thumb and the radial two and a half fingers is the classical pattern. However, it is common for patients to localize paraesthesia atypically. Keenan (1991) found that only 38% of 103 patients with confirmed carpal tunnel

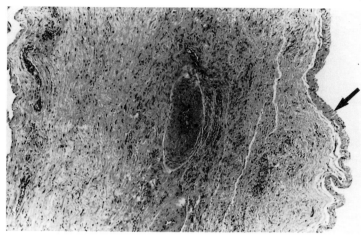

Figure 5.18 The typical histological features of thickened synovium in carpal tunnel syndrome, showing fibrosis, hypervascularity and compact collagenosis (*arrow*) beneath the surface coating of flattened synovial cells. There is also a scanty lymphocytic infiltrate and an increase in plump active fibroblasts. There is considerable variation in degree of thickening of the synovium in carpal tunnel syndrome; this example is severe. Despite the absence of the typical changes of inflammation, in carpal tunnel syndrome symptomatic improvement is often achieved by injection of steroid into the tunnel. (Courtesy A. Stevens, Department of Histopathology, University Hospital, Nottingham)

syndrome described paraesthesia in the cutaneous distribution of the median nerve; the fifth finger was involved in 30% and the whole hand in 20%.

The symptoms are usually worse at night, but discomfort, burning, tingling and numbness may all be apparent diurnally. Discomfort may radiate proximally to the forearm, upper arm, shoulder and neck, possibly as a result of peripheral or central sensitization of the nervous system. Under these circumstances, tenderness of the nerve may be detected in the arm. An alternative explanation for axially orientated symptoms is coincidental cervical (or proximal thoracic) spinal joint dysfunction and/or nerve root irritation.

Although sensory symptoms are predominant initially, motor function may be affected in the more chronic case. Complaints of numbness, clumsiness and weakness of pinch and grip are not unusual at a later stage, the symptoms arising from weakness of opposition of the thumb in addition to loss of coordination and sensory disturbance.

Occasionally, evidence of autonomic dysfunction or sympathetic overactivity is seen. Kopell and Thompson (1963) consider that involvement of the autonomic nervous system is extremely common. Sometimes this manifests as a diffuse discoloration with alteration in sweating; at other times, blanching suggestive of Raynaud's phenomenon may be seen.

In summary, acknowledging that electrodiagnostic tests are not 100% reliable in the early case (see below), patients' symptomatology assumes considerable diagnostic importance. The combination of neuritic symptoms in the median nerve distribution, their nocturnal intensification and the need to hang the affected arm out of bed at night to seek relief is virtually pathognomonic of CTS. When the symptoms are not characteristic, further positive evidence, clinical or electrodiagnostic, is required.

Examination findings

The diagnosis of CTS often presents few difficulties when the history is 'classical' and when Phalen's test or the Tinel sign are positive. When the history is atypical, however, complete reliance upon the provocation tests is unwise. Katz *et al.* (1990) reported that the sensitivity of Phalen's test is only 75%, and the sensitivity of the percussion test (Tinel sign) is even worse, at 60%. These findings are generally in accord with most observers' experiences. Kuschner *et al.* (1992) have demonstrated from their own series of control patients (endorsed by a study of the literature) that the specificity of the Tinel test is poor – little better than 50% (indicating a high false-positive rate). They concluded that Tinel's test could not be recommended but that both the sensitivity and specificity of Phalen's test are greater.

Even when Tinel's test is performed by the application of firm pressure, rather than tapping, over the transverse carpal ligament, the test is unreliable (probably due to the loss of transmission of forces to the median nerve on account of the thickness of the ligament). However, increased sensitivity (79% according to Mossman and Blau, 1989) may result from the use of a broad-based 'Queen Square' tendon hammer to percuss the volar aspect of the extended wrist.

Phalen (1966) reported that prompt relief after injection of a steroid into the carpal tunnel gives additional support to the diagnosis. In my view, the diagnostic usefulness of an intra-carpal tunnel injection cannot be overstressed.

Disturbed motor function and/or thenar atrophy are late signs of CTS, and should not be awaited for the purpose of diagnosis. When present, the motor signs are weakness of abduction and/or weakness of opposition of the thumb.

Hypoaesthesia becomes apparent and clumsiness with buttons may be observed as the condition progresses. In the early stages, however, hyperaesthesiae in the distribution of the median nerve may be experienced. When positive, two point discrimination tests indicate advanced nerve dysfunction. Tenderness along the line of the median nerve may be detected in the forearm. Occasionally, swelling of the flexor tendon complex at the volar aspect of the wrist may be found. This, of course, indicates the probability that flexor tenosynovitis is the cause of the CTS.

The cervical spine should be examined in patients with arm pain or dysaesthesia, even if the symptoms are typical of a specific peripheral nerve entrapment. This is particularly important in suspected lesions of the median nerve or ulnar nerve. The symptoms of carpal tunnel syndrome may be mimicked by C6 or C7 nerve root irritation. There is poor correlation between root compression/irritation and the presence of spinal degenerative changes on X-ray, hence the need for a comprehensive examination of the cervical spine, including neural tension tests, as described in Chapter 7.

Nerve conduction studies are often undertaken, but are fraught with potential pitfalls (Szabo and Madison, 1992), including operator dependency and standardization of normal values. The 'classic' finding is *prolonged distal wrist latency* in conduction velocity, particularly on sensory as opposed to motor conduction tests. The segment of nerve from palm to wrist shows the lowest velocity, and this may be the only detectable abnormality (Mills, 1985). However, normal electrophysiological tests are often found in early cases of CTS, even when sensory action potentials are recorded from stimulation of the palmar branch of the median nerve.

Median nerve neuropathy may exist in a subclinical state until a relevant stress provokes sufficient nerve damage for it to become symptomatic. This may explain the widespread prevalence (39% of all subjects) of impaired sensory conduction of the median nerve in a random sample of manual workers across four industries (Nathan *et al.*, 1988). Symptomatology was not recorded.

As with other clinical tests, a lack of confirmatory evidence (an absence of electrophysiological abnormalities in this instance) should not be considered to refute the diagnosis. It is worthy of note that nerve conduction studies are performed during the operator's working day, whereas the patient's symptoms are often predominantly nocturnal.

Finally, the diagnosis of CTS should always be accompanied by a general examination of the patient to exclude systemic ('constitutional') as well as local causes. In particular, hypothyroidism, diabetes, rheumatoid arthritis and peripheral neuritis (associated with alcoholism for instance) should be considered. Local to the wrist, radiocarpal osteoarthritis and swellings such as ganglions, lipomas and neuromas should be excluded. Clinical features that suggest the development of a type 2 work-related upper limb disorder as a consequence of median nerve compression are not unusual; allodynia and hyperalgesia are usually meaningful clinical signs, and should be recorded.

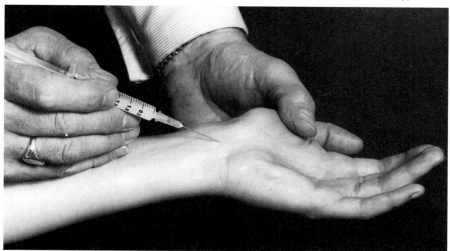

Figure 5.19 Injection of the carpal tunnel is demonstrated. The injection site is just proximal to the distal wrist crease, approximately mid-way between the pisiform bone and the tubercle of the scaphoid. The needle penetrates at approximately 45 degrees to the plane of the forearm

Management

Underlying medical conditions should be treated. In the absence of systemic conditions, and when CTS is caused by or aggravated by work factors, patients should be advised to discuss their complaints with their employers. In the early stages resolution of CTS may be achieved by reduction of provocative activities alone. Night splinting is often helpful if a conservative regimen is instituted. The use of non-steroidal anti-inflammatory medication is logical, particularly when there is flexor tendinitis, but the response is often disappointing.

Injection of steroid into the carpal tunnel usually gives relief, but this too should be combined with a radical assessment of work activities to prevent recurrence. Injection of 5–10 mg of triamcinolone (combined optionally with 1 ml of 1% lignocaine) in a 2 ml syringe fitted with a 23 gauge needle is sufficient. The patient's wrist is maintained in approximately 30 degrees of dorsiflexion and a point is chosen 0.5–1.0 cm proximal to the distal wrist crease, approximately mid-way between the pisiform bone and the tubercle of the scaphoid (Figure 5.19). This is usually just to the radial side of palmaris longus when present. The needle penetrates at approximately 45 degrees to the plane of the forearm. The injection should require modest pressure only on the plunger of the syringe.

Transient numbness or paraesthesiae may be experienced after the injection but, if slight, are not of any concern, and the patient informed accordingly. However, as median nerve palsy has been caused by intraneural injection, the needle should be adjusted if paraesthesiae are experienced at the start of the injection. For maximum safety, infiltration may be made following placement of the needle to the ulnar side of palmaris longus.

Gelberman *et al.* (1988) reported on the success of intracarpal tunnel steroid injections followed by splinting for three weeks in a high percentage of cases. However, at 18 months, less than 50% of the mild cases and less than 25% of the more severe cases remained asymptomatic. The injection may be repeated after a few weeks if there has been a partial response, but recurrence of symptoms indicates the need for surgery.

Decompression of the carpal tunnel by section of the transverse carpal ligament is usually successful, and may allow the patient to return to a job requiring repetitive hand actions. Numerous surgical series have confirmed the generally excellent results of surgery (Rosenbaum and Ochoa, 1993). Semple and Cargill (1969) reported 75% of hands asymptomatic at follow-up 2–7 years after surgery (and 97% excellent results in those patients with symptoms for less than 6 months). Other authors have quoted up to 99% of hands improved). Phalen (1966) found that 77% of patients who had impaired sensation prior to surgery for CTS recovered normal sensation.

Nevertheless, surgery is not without complications, despite their infrequency. Postoperative reflex sympathetic dystrophy is uncommon, and the risk is lessened by limiting surgery to those with clear electrodiagnostic confirmation. When reflex sympathetic dystrophy occurs the resultant disability is usually profound. Damage to the palmar cutaneous nerve may occur. Scars may become hypertrophic or tender. However, it is probable that the majority of poor results (as reflected by the persistence of symptoms) are not due to inadequate decompression, but are caused by the failure to recognize concurrent cervical nerve root irritation or the development of neuropathic arm pain, with only a minor contribution to symptoms from the precipitating median nerve compression.

The pronator syndrome

The median nerve may be subject to entrapment during its passage through the pronator teres muscle in the proximal forearm (Figure 5.20). Kopell and Thompson (1963) state that in this region the most likely cause of entrapment is hypertrophy of the pronator teres muscle secondary to repeated forceful pronation of the forearm accompanied by forceful finger flexion. Such activities are seen on the assembly line and in some sports such as vigorous serving at tennis. Musicians are a particularly vulnerable group because of the frequent repetitive pronation required (Bejjani *et al.*, 1996).

Howard (1986) has identified a number of other possibilities: a sharp lacertus fibrosus (the broad aponeurotic expansion of the distal biceps), a sharp edge to flexor digitorum sublimis, a fibrous band (for instance a thickened ligament of Struthers) or a supracondylar bony spur. Direct trauma to the antecubital fossa and proximal volar forearm is a very occasional cause of acute pronator syndrome.

Both sensory and motor manifestations may arise. The sensory disturbances in the hand are in the same distribution as with CTS, with the addition of an extended palmar component. In addition to weakness of grasp, the

loss of muscle power in the wrist and finger flexors leads to clumsy, awkward movements of the thumb and fingers.

The differentiating features of pronator syndrome when compared to CTS are: exacerbation of sensory symptoms by pressure over the median nerve in the forearm (whereas in CTS the nerve is tender only); extension of sensory impairment to the radial palm as well as the thumb and radial fingers; increased pain on resisted forearm pronation or wrist flexion (which should be differentiated from medial epicondylitis by other features and additional tests); more extensive motor weakness, but less thenar atrophy in the late cases. Electrophysiological tests should also differentiate from carpal tunnel syndrome.

Local infiltration of steroid and local anaesthetic may be used diagnostically as well as therapeutically. In the refractory case, surgical exploration is necessary.

The anterior interosseous syndrome

The anterior interosseous nerve arises from the median nerve 5–8 cm distal to the antecubital fossa. It innervates the flexor pollicis longus, the radial half of the flexor digitorum profundus and the pronator quadratus.

Local trauma or hypertrophy of the pronator teres are the more common causes of entrapment neuropathy in which the loss of normal pinch is a characteristic feature. Weakness of flexion of the terminal digit of the index finger and of the thumb are associated with abnormal pulp contact (Spinner, 1970). As pronator teres is unaffected, loss of active pronation of the forearm is partial. Weakness is more profound in elbow flexion, when pronator teres is relatively ineffective.

In the absence of spontaneous recovery over 2–3 months, surgical exploration is advisable.

The ulnar nerve

Distal ulnar nerve entrapment

The ulnar nerve enters the hand through Guyon's canal, a shallow trough between the pisiform and hamate bones (Figure 5.21). The

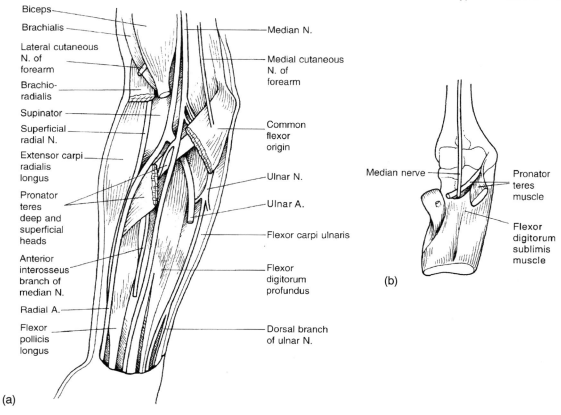

Figure 5.20 (*a*) The median nerve or its branch, the anterior interosseous nerve, may be compressed during its passage through the pronator teres muscle. (After H. Ellis and S. Feldman, *Anatomy for Anaesthetists*, Blackwell, Oxford, 1993) (*b*) A sharp edge to flexor digitorum sublimis may impinge upon the median nerve. (After Kopell and Thompson, 1963)

canal runs distally for approximately 1.5 cm from the distal flexion crease of the wrist; its roof is an aponeurotic extension of the flexor carpi ulnaris tendon and the overlying palmaris brevis muscle. The ulnar nerve divides into deep and superficial branches in the region of the pisiform bone. The deep branch passes between the abductor digiti minimi and flexor digiti minimi muscles, innervating the interossei, the ulnar lumbricals and adductor pollicis as well as the muscles of the hypothenar eminence. The superficial branch is sensory, supplying the skin over the hypothenar eminence and the palmar surface of the ulnar one and a half digits. Variably, a dorsal cutaneous (sensory) nerve is given off by the ulnar nerve above the wrist, in which case the sensation to the dorsal ulnar aspect of

the hand is spared in the presence of a lesion in Guyon's canal.

In Guyon's canal a neuropathy may arise from repeated compression of the main trunk of the nerve or its superficial branch by the use of hand-held tools such as screwdrivers and pliers. Some assembly jobs also require repetitive forceful striking of the palm against relatively immovable objects. A handlebar palsy may occur in cyclists as a result of constant pressure on the pisiform and adjacent tissues by dropped handlebars. Occasionally, neuropraxia may be caused by isolated trauma, for instance the forceful use of the heel of the hand to open a sash window (Kopell and Thompson, 1963).

Space-occupying lesions such as ganglia or synovial proliferation in rheumatoid arthritis

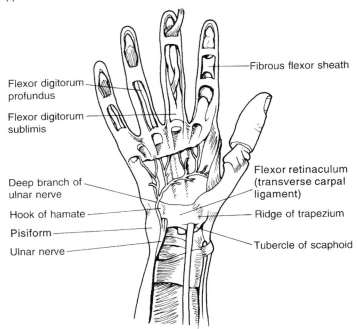

Flexor digitorum profundus

Flexor digitorum sublimis

Deep branch of ulnar nerve

Hook of hamate

Pisiform

Ulnar nerve

Fibrous flexor sheath

Flexor retinaculum (transverse carpal ligament)

Ridge of trapezium

Tubercle of scaphoid

Figure 5.21 The ulnar nerve may be compressed in Guyon's canal, a shallow trough between the pisiform and hamate bones

may cause pressure on the deep branch of the ulnar nerve.

The presenting complaints are dependent upon whether the main trunk, the superficial branch or the deep branch is the site of entrapment. For instance, distal compression may affect the first dorsal interosseus but spare the abductor digiti minini on clinical testing. Burning pain and sensory disturbances in the ulnar one and a half digits are caused by compression of the main trunk and its superficial branch. Hyperaesthesia may precede hypoaesthesia. Compression of the motor component gives rise to weakness of the small muscles of the hand; weakness of the hypothenar muscles is usually obvious clinically. Patients may complain of weakness of pinch because of the loss of power of adductor pollicis.

Nerve conduction studies are necessary to identify the site of entrapment as accurately as possible, and to differentiate the problem from the cubital tunnel syndrome. Soft tissue scanning techniques may be helpful to identify a space-occupying lesion.

Localized steroid and local anaesthetic injections may be therapeutic in the less well-

established case. Otherwise, surgical exploration is necessary, particularly if there is a suspicion of a space-occupying lesion.

The cubital tunnel syndrome

The ulnar nerve is at risk in the ulnar groove (the cubital tunnel) behind the medial epicondyle at the elbow as a consequence of its superficial position. It may be traumatized during a specific incident – for instance a blow to the posteromedial aspect of the elbow – or by repetitive compression. The latter situation commonly arises when the elbow rests against a firm surface during manual activities such as handwriting.

The ulnar nerve may be compressed at the elbow by a thickened aponeurosis of the flexor carpi ulnaris as the nerve enters the forearm between the two heads of the muscle (Howard, 1986) (Figure 5.22). The dimensions of the cubital tunnel are compromised further by elbow flexion. Other causative factors are osteophytic outgrowths, fibrosis secondary to tensile and valgus forces to the medial elbow in baseball pitchers, field athletes and tennis players, a large carrying angle (cubitus valgus

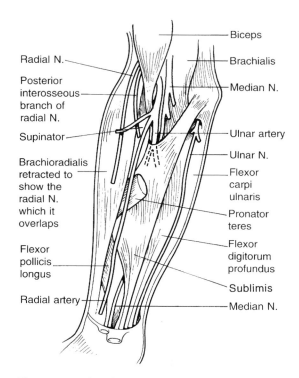

Radial N.

Posterior interosseous branch of radial N.

Supinator

Brachioradialis retracted to show the radial N. which it overlaps

Flexor pollicis longus

Radial artery

Biceps

Brachialis

Median N.

Ulnar artery

Ulnar N.

Flexor carpi ulnaris

Pronator teres

Flexor digitorum profundus

Sublimis

Median N.

Figure 5.22 The ulnar nerve may be compressed by a thickened aponeurosis of the flexor carpi ulnaris as the nerve enters the forearm between the two heads of the muscle

– which probably increases the tautness of the nerve in the ulnar groove) and recurrent dislocation of the nerve from its groove. However, in some cases no such predisposing causes can be identified.

Dysaesthesiae – burning and hyperaesthesiae – in the fourth and fifth digits are early symptoms. Subsequently numbness and loss of motor power are experienced. The typical picture of complete ulnar palsy is well documented in orthopaedic and neurological texts: the weakness of the intrinsic hand muscles causes hyperextension at the MCP joints and flexion at the IP joints to give the 'claw' hand; there is hypothenar and interosseous wasting. When the neuropathy arises as a 'late' consequence of an injury, the term 'tardy ulnar palsy' is sometimes applied.

Symptoms may radiate proximally, usually along the inner aspect of the upper arm, mimicking C8 or T1 root compression. The differential diagnosis includes the thoracic outlet syndrome (in which T1 root symptoms are predominant, often bilaterally), C8 root

entrapment in the neck, T3 syndrome (Fraser, 1990), and neuropathic arm pain (which may be a secondary consequence of ulnar nerve irritation/entrapment).

Nerve conduction studies are necessary to confirm the site of entrapment neuropathy. X-rays of the elbow that demonstrate the cubital tunnel are required to detect intrusive osteophytes.

Management is dependent upon the identification of the cause of the cubital tunnel syndrome. Simple measures such as the avoidance of pressure on the posteromedial aspect of the elbow(s) at work may suffice in some cases but surgery is normally required to avoid progressive deterioration in hand function. Surgical decompression may be necessary if there is intrinsic mechanical compression. Anterior transposition of the ulnar nerve is an alternative surgical strategy, particularly for the hypermobile ulnar nerve.

Foster and Edshage (1981) obtained 92% improvement following surgical management of cases of ulnar nerve entrapment. Cubital decompression and anterior subcutaneous transposition of the ulnar nerve gave equally good results in the relief of the symptoms of pain and dysaesthesia. However, anterior transposition was more effective with respect to the recovery of motor function.

The radial nerve

Radial tunnel syndrome

Epidemiology/aetiology

Radial nerve entrapment has been described in some detail by Kopell and Thompson (1963) and by Roles and Maudsley (1972). It may arise as a result of localized direct trauma or (more usually) by overuse of the adjacent muscle groups. Kopell and Thompson identified repeated forceful supination, wrist dorsiflexion or radial deviation against resistance as aetiological factors; thus, the condition may arise in tennis players (from the stresses associated with backhand shots) or in workers using a heavy hammer, for instance. Roles and Maudsley found that half of their patients subjected to surgery for this condition had occupations that required repetitive pronation/supination or forceful wrist extension

– such as bricklayers, fitters, machine operators and telephonists.

Pathoanatomy

In the upper arm the radial nerve winds its way downwards from the medial to the lateral side of the humerus (where it may be compressed in 'Saturday night palsy'). At the elbow the nerve pierces the lateral intermuscular septum to lie in front of the capitellum of the humerus between the brachialis and brachioradialis muscles (the start of the radial tunnel). It becomes intimately associated anatomically with the anterior aspect of the radial head where it divides into the deep motor branch (subsequently to become the posterior interosseous nerve) and the superficial sensory branch.

The deep branch passes under the edge (described by Kopell and Thompson as 'fibrous') of the extensor carpi radialis brevis muscle which has an extensive origin stretching from the lateral epicondyle to the deep fascia overlying the supinator muscle. It pierces the supinator muscle (Figure 5.23; see also Figure 7.24) to wind laterally around the neck of the radius and subsequently to lie adjacent to the interosseous membrane during its descent down the posterior aspect of the forearm – where it is known as the posterior interosseous nerve. It is a motor nerve innervating the wrist and finger dorsiflexors.

The deep branch of the radial nerve may be entrapped by tightening of the fibrous edge of the extensor carpi radialis brevis (Kopell and Thompson). Roles and Maudsley, on the other hand, considered that 'resistant tennis elbow' was caused by radial nerve entrapment in the radial tunnel by the arcade of Frohse – the thickened or fibrotic superior edge of the supinator.

Clinical features

The clinical features are similar to 'classic' tennis elbow. Patients complain of pain, tenderness and weakness of grip (principally as a result of pain inhibition). Occasionally, paraesthesiae in the distribution of the superficial radial nerve are experienced. The examination findings are often identical to those of lateral epicondylitis: pain on passive stretching of the wrist and finger extensors and pain on isometric contraction. Roles and Maudsley emphasized the diagnostic importance of resisted extension of the middle finger with the elbow extended, but this test is usually positive in lateral epicondylitis too.

It is my experience that there are two examination features that should raise the possibility of nerve entrapment rather than enthesitis: pain (and weakness in the established case) on resisted supination of the forearm, and tenderness over the radial head. Although impaired motor function may also manifest as wasting and weakness of the wrist and finger extensors, these signs are unusual. Nerve conduction studies may be positive. The diagnosis is most often made retrospectively when there has been poor response to localized steroid and local anaesthetic injections for a presumptive diagnosis of lateral epicondylitis.

Management

Once the diagnosis has been established, surgical dissection and division of constricting fibrous tissues, such as the arcade of Frohse, gives good results in the vast majority of patients (Roles and Maudsley). Localized infiltration of local anaesthetic and steroid has a useful role diagnostically, but more radical treatment should not be delayed in the presence of positive signs and failure of conservative management.

Superficial radial neuropathy ('Wartenberg's syndrome')

The superficial branch of the radial nerve remains superficial to the extensor carpi radialis, descending into the forearm beneath brachioradialis. On emerging from brachioradialis, the nerve winds around the radius, pierces the deep fascia and becomes subcutaneous (Figures 5.9a, 5.24), where it is most vulnerable to trauma. It is a sensory nerve, innervating the skin over the radial side of the dorsum of the wrist and hand, terminating as the dorsal digital nerves to the radial three and a half digits.

Compression of the superficial sensory branch of the radial nerve above the wrist was described by Wartenberg (1932), who coined the term 'cheiralgia paraesthetica'. The early cases were thought to have arisen as a result

(a)

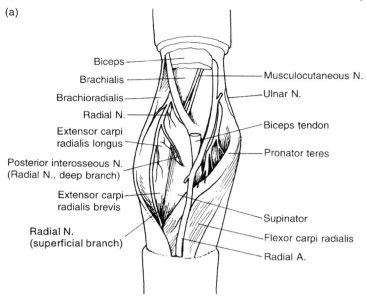

- Biceps
- Brachialis
- Brachioradialis
- Radial N.
- Extensor carpi radialis longus
- Posterior interosseous N. (Radial N., deep branch)
- Extensor carpi radialis brevis
- Radial N. (superficial branch)

- Musculocutaneous N.
- Ulnar N.
- Biceps tendon
- Pronator teres
- Supinator
- Flexor carpi radialis
- Radial A.

(b)

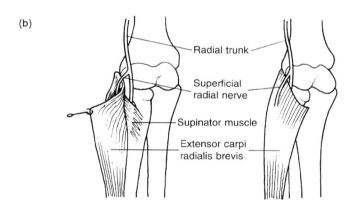

- Radial trunk
- Superficial radial nerve
- Supinator muscle
- Extensor carpi radialis brevis

Figure 5.23 The posterior interosseous nerve (the deep branch of the radial nerve) may be entrapped (*a*) by the arcade of Frohse (the thickened superior edge of the supinator muscle) or (*b*) by the fibrous edge of the extensor carpi radialis brevis

of a tight wrist-watch strap. Other identified causes have included the use of handcuffs or splints, and operations around the wrist.

When the nerve is traumatized, paraesthesiae affect the radial border of the distal forearm and the base of the thumb. Tinel's sign was positive in all twelve cases in a series described by Braidwood (1975). In the context of occupational disorders it has been hypothesized that repetitive 'stretching' of the nerve (by ulnar deviation of the wrist combined with flexion of the thumb) may be an aetiological factor. Whatever the cause, the condition is uncommon in clinical practice.

Reflex sympathetic dystrophy (RSD) (syn. algodystrophy, Sudeck's atrophy)

Although the term RSD was not coined until some fifty years ago (Evans, 1947), the condition, in one form or another, has been recognized for much longer. The large number of

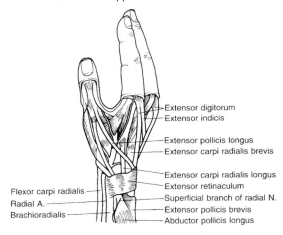

Extensor digitorum
Extensor indicis

Extensor pollicis longus
Extensor carpi radialis brevis

Extensor carpi radialis longus
Extensor retinaculum

Flexor carpi radialis
Radial A.
Brachioradialis

Superficial branch of radial N.
Extensor pollicis brevis
Abductor pollicis longus

Figure 5.24 The superficial branch of the radial nerve is vulnerable to trauma in the distal forearm. The tendons over the radial aspect of the wrist are illustrated

synonyms (of which only two are given above) and the diverse methods of approach to management reflect the complexity of the condition – or groups of disorders – and its refractoriness to treatment.

RSD is characterized by pain, dysaesthesiae, vasomotor and sudomotor abnormalities, abnormalities of the motor system, and trophic changes in both superficial and deep tissues (Herrick, 1994). The sympathetic nervous system appears to play an important role in the development and perpetuation of the condition; this hypothesis is reinforced by the response, albeit only temporary in some instances, to sympathetic blockade. Its relationship to other WRULDs or to work activities in general may be marginal (or 'end stage' in some cases), but there are a number of factors in common with other conditions affecting the upper limb.

Epidemiology and aetiology
RSD may affect either the upper or lower limb; sometimes it is bilateral. It usually arises as a consequence of trauma (with or without an obvious nerve injury), and less commonly after visceral diseases (such as the shoulder/hand syndrome after myocardial infarction), or after central nervous system lesions (such as brain injury). Occasionally, it is idiopathic.

As the relatively minor form (see below) is probably underdiagnosed, it is likely that the

incidence is probably considerably higher than the estimation of one case in 2000 accidents involving an extremity (Plewes, 1956). In the upper limb, RSD may be considered to represent an exaggerated response to a painful event, commonly trauma (including surgery).

Pathophysiology
It is postulated that the initiating event/trauma provokes a significant sympathetic discharge in addition to nociceptor activation. Sensitization of peripheral afferent neurones and alteration of central nervous system processing are responsible for widespread allodynia. Fuelled by sympathetic activity, further nociceptor and low-threshold mechanoreceptor stimulation causes a vicious cycle of pain and reflex responses to develop (Janig, 1990). Abnormalities of the sweating mechanism and disturbances of peripheral blood flow lead to raised interstitial pressures and trophic changes.

RSD may be viewed as having two associations with WRULDs. Both RSD and type 2 WRULD have underlying neurogenic mechanisms; and RSD may arise as a consequence of a type 1 WRULD (but usually as a result of specific trauma such as surgery for carpal tunnel syndrome or peripheral nerve injury).

Clinical features
Pain is the predominant symptom; it is constant and diffuse, and is frequently described as burning in quality. This type of pain, in combination with marked allodynia, is almost pathognomonic of a neurogenic aetiology. The significance of the non-dermatomal distribution of pain and hyperaesthesiae may be misinterpreted clinically, encouraging the development or perpetuation of abnormal illness behaviour (which is a common accompaniment of RSD).

The extremities are primarily affected. When the upper limb is affected the pain usually begins in the hand and wrist, but may spread proximally. The subjective response to the severe allodynia and hyperpathia is the early withdrawal of the hand and arm from normal use.

Examination findings
Guarding of the affected part is usually observed, and may be severe. Patients often

prefer to keep the forearm and hand immobile in a sling, and are reluctant to have the hand examined. The examination findings, in particular the clinical manifestations of the sudomotor and vasomotor changes, are dependent upon the stage of the condition. Although three stages are often described, it is useful from a management standpoint to classify RSD as 'early' and 'established'.

Early The vasomotor changes are predominantly *vasodilatory*. The extremity is usually warm, red or mottled, and hyperhydrotic. Accelerated growth of hair on the forearm is often seen. There is tissue oedema and extensive allodynia and hyperpathia. Movements of the wrist and fingers are performed very slowly and carefully by the patient. This stage merges insidiously with the established case as vasoconstriction and dystrophic changes gradually occur.

Established Pain continues and becomes more diffuse. As a result of reduced dermal blood flow in this *vasoconstrictive* stage, the extremity gradually becomes cool, and the skin assumes a characteristic pale and atrophic appearance. Dystrophic changes occur in the nails, and contractures at the MCP and IP joints are observed. Allodynia and hyperpathia persist. In the advanced case the hand progressively loses function for other than very coarse manoeuvres, and proximal disturbances manifest as progressive immobility at the shoulder as a result of a capsulitis that is indistinguishable from frozen shoulder. Despite the gross loss of function the patient may develop a curious indifference to their useless limb.

The features of the early case are usually present for some months; progression is not invariable, but when contractures occur these are usually irreversible. Eventually, pain diminishes but permanent disability may be profound.

Investigations
Once RSD is established, X-rays reveal patchy osteoporosis of the affected extremity. Radionuclide bone scanning reveals increased uptake at an earlier stage (Figure 5.25). Thermography may assist, but remains principally a research tool. Predominantly, RSD should be a clinical diagnosis requiring a high index of

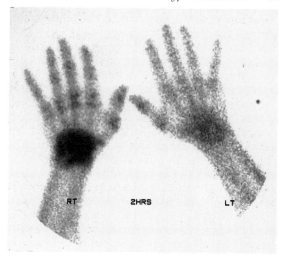

Figure 5.25 Radionuclide scan in the bone phase taken 2 hours after injection, showing increased uptake in the right wrist and hand. The involvement of all the joints, including the metacarpal and interphalangeal joints as well as the carpus, is typical of reflex sympathetic dystrophy

suspicion on the part of the clinician. In comparison with other work-related upper limb disorders, the autonomic nervous system activity is the distinguishing characteristic.

Management
The results of treatment of the early stage of RSD are probably vastly superior to the management of the established case. Even so, the results are largely anecdotal.

It is generally accepted that **active exercise** of the affected limb in patients with the early features of RSD after traumatic injury is the keystone of treatment, to overcome the fear of pain and to regain function. Hence, the importance of clinical awareness and early diagnosis. Passive exercises should be undertaken by a skilled physiotherapist. Gentle mobilization may be necessary initially as untimely overenthusiasm may exacerbate the condition in a limb that already exhibits allodynia and hyperpathia. For similar reasons the extremes of heat and cold may be tolerated badly. Generally, the combination of mobilization exercises and encouragement is often successful in the early case in which there are few, if any, dystrophic changes. At this stage, if progress is not being made, **sympathetic blockade** must be carried out (see below).

Advancement to the well-established stage offers a relatively poor prognosis. (Spontaneous remission in a minority of cases only is observed.) Although sympathetic blockade is considered by many pain specialists to be the treatment of choice, its success is somewhat dependent upon treatment commencing within 6 months of the onset of symptoms. Regional blockade is usually performed by intravenous guanethidine blocks, using a Bier's block technique. Alternatively, one or more paravertebral sympathetic blocks, for instance to the stellate ganglion (or to the lumbar sympathetic chain for lower limb pain), may be helpful. Epidural blocks have been tried, and are successful in some cases, but symptomatic relief is usually only temporary. Oral steroid therapy has been reported to give good results, but is used much less frequently than sympathetic blocks. TENS pain relief is often a useful adjunct.

FOCAL DYSTONIA

Occupational disorders affecting the hand, characterized by 'cramps', involuntary movements or loss of normal control, have been recognized since the beginning of the eighteenth century (Ramazzini, 1713). Lederman (1991), in a review of the literature, noted that occupational cramp in a pianist was reported by Romberg in 1853, and in a flautist by Bianchi in 1878. The condition of writer's cramp or 'scrivener's palsy' was described in great detail by authors such as Gowers (1883) and Poore (1887) towards the end of the nineteenth century. Poore described the condition of 'piano failure' in 21 pianists, associating it with similar conditions found in other occupations, collectively known as occupational cramp, craft or occupational palsy, or occupational neurosis.

Occupational cramp of the hand is a prescribed disease (PD A4) in the UK. According to the Social Security (Industrial Injuries) (Prescribed Diseases) Regulations, 1975 the occupations in which this arises are prolonged periods of handwriting, typing or other repetitive movements of the fingers, hand or arm.

The term 'dystonia' was first used by Oppenheim in 1911 but it has not been until the past twenty years or so that the concept of occupational cramp as a form of focal dystonia has evolved. The condition has been researched primarily at those centres specializing in musicians' injuries.

The working definition proposed by Lederman (1988) is that 'dystonia is a syndrome of sustained or, at least initially, intermittent muscle contractions, frequently causing twisting and repetitive movements or abnormal postures'. The characteristic abnormality is simultaneous (co-)contraction of agonist and antagonist muscles, occurring in task-specific activities. One or more fingers are usually affected, though in no definite pattern. Men are more frequently affected than women.

In Lederman's series of more than 500 instrumentalists with 'professionally related problems', 8% suffered from focal dystonia. In wind players the muscles forming the embouchure (the position of the lips) may be affected. The lack of progression of musician's cramp (and occupational cramp or writer's cramp), the task-specificity and the lack of family history distinguish focal dystonia from the larger group of progressive dystonias.

The most common complaint in musicians (for instance violinists and pianists) is impaired control or dexterity (Hochberg *et al.*, 1983; Lederman, 1988; Newmark and Hochberg, 1987). Stiffness, cramp, tightness and excessive fatigue are further symptoms. Pain is an unusual feature. The precipitating activity is commonly excessive playing, though a change in technique may also be causal. Task-specificity may not be absolute, as there may be a cross-reference to writing or typing skills, but instrumentalists who play more than one instrument find that the condition affects the playing of one instrument only. Sometimes symptoms may be ameliorated by certain manoeuvres or 'sensory (proprioceptive) tricks', for instance touching the writing hand with one finger of the opposite hand. However, the improvement is only temporary.

The diagnosis depends upon an adequate description of the condition by the patient, or (preferably) the observation of the motor dystonia by the examiner, and the absence of other neuromuscular abnormalities. In particular, a neuropathy must be excluded: for instance, compensatory movements in patients with a minor degree of motor weakness due to ulnar nerve entrapment may mimic the involuntary muscle contractions exhibited by patients with a focal dystonia. The condition must also be differentiated from other forms of dystonia, for instance those associated with neurological conditions.

The multitude of therapeutic strategies that are frequently applied to focal dystonia is testimony to the lack of understanding of the pathophysiology. The protagonists of psychotherapy, physical modalities, behavioural techniques and complete rest offer anecdotal evidence for their efficacy in a modest percentage of patients only. The relearning of playing techniques, combined with slow practice, has been the mainstay of treatment in most musicians' clinics. The use of botulinum toxin, which appears to offer hope of more rapid control of symptoms in a significant percentage of patients, has emerged as an alternative treatment in experienced hands (Cohen *et al.*, 1987).

SHOULDER PAIN

Shoulder pain is a common burden in occupations that demand repetitive use of the hand and arm, particularly when the arm is moved away from the side of the body and the hands reach to shoulder height. The differential diagnosis often includes both primary shoulder conditions and secondary manifestations of problems originating elsewhere.

The evaluation of the aetiology and diagnosis of shoulder pain requires an awareness by the clinician of the relationship between cervical spinal dysfunction and subacromial dysfunction. Diagnostic difficulties may arise as the result of the frequent use of the term 'shoulder' by patients whose discomfort may be felt anteriorly, posteriorly, laterally or superiorly in the shoulder region.

The following account is an attempt to evaluate some of the conditions that may be work-related and which give rise to discomfort or pain around the shoulder and in the upper arm. Subacromial disturbances may arise as a result of:

(a) functional disturbances at the subacromial joint (subacromial dysfunction);

(b) pathoanatomical changes at the subacromial 'joint' (subacromial impingement).

These will be described in some detail. Secondary hyperalgesia too, particularly scapular but also subclavicular, may be manifest around the shoulder, and is discussed further under Myofascial pain.

Subacromial dysfunction

The relationship between dysfunction in the lower cervical or proximal thoracic spine and subacromial dysfunction is poorly understood. Undoubtedly, shoulder pain and the clinical signs of subacromial dysfunction (particularly a painful arc on abduction of the arm) are commonly associated with disturbances in the cervical spine. This association is the more likely when discomfort radiates from the neck to the upper arm. When a thorough examination is conducted, a *triad* of signs is commonly found – positive neural tension, subacromial dysfunction and a myofascial trigger point in the proximal scapular fixator muscles – in addition to the local signs of somatic (segmental) spinal dysfunction. Under these circumstances, subacromial dysfunction may be a manifestation of mechanical hyperalgesia.

Subacromial impingement

The diagnosis of subacromial impingement is commonly predicated upon traumatic, degenerative or inflammatory changes in the subacromial soft tissues.

Pathoanatomy
The underlying pathology is usually rotator cuff disease which may be classified according to its progression (Brox *et al.*, 1993): acute inflammation – tendinitis (stage 1); degeneration – chronic tendinosis (stage 2); rupture (stage 3). Subacromial bursitis is commonly associated with any stage of the disease.

An acute tendinitis results from overload. The supraspinatus tendon is the most commonly affected as a result of repetitive abduction of the arm(s) or maintenance of the arms in an abducted position. The infraspinatus tendon and the subscapularis tendon may also be affected. Although the biceps brachii tendon is not strictly part of the rotator cuff, bicipital tendinitis too may result from unaccustomed or repetitive use of the arm.

Rotator cuff tendinosis, on the other hand, is basically degenerative, resulting from and being accelerated by repetitive use (Figure 5.26). Pathological changes in the rotator cuff have been attributed to primary mechanical impingement, for instance from inferior osteophytes at an osteoarthritic acromioclavicular joint (Hutson, 1996) (Figure 5.27). Alternatively, degeneration may result from ischaemia in the hypovascular region, noted by Rathbun and MacNab (1970) to be centred in the tendinous portion of the supraspinatus proximal to its insertion into the greater tuberosity. Whatever the pathogenesis of rotator cuff tendinosis, a consequence is the development of a chronic fibrotic subacromial bursitis which causes significant disturbance to subacromial function. A self-perpetuating cycle of bursitis and tendinitis/tendinosis is caused by impingement of the soft tissues under the acromion and the tough coracoacromial ligament. Heterotopic calcification too may arise as part of the degenerative process, contributing further to mechanical impingement (Figure 5.28).

Substantive injuries to the rotator cuff, for instance a partial or complete tear, may arise as a result of a fall on to the shoulder, a sudden wrenching of the shoulder, or a relatively minor strain if the cuff is already degenerate (Figure 5.29). Most commonly, the injury is to the supraspinatus tendon, which forms the floor of the subacromial 'joint'. A rotator cuff tear acts as a space-occupying lesion, giving rise to disturbed subacromial function.

Epidemiology and aetiology

Rotator cuff tendinitis results from excessive demands upon the tendon, irrespective of whether its premorbid morphological state was normal or whether it was degenerate. Repeated or sustained abduction of the shoulders may be a prominent feature of sporting, domestic or recreational activities. The use of hedge clippers may provoke the condition in gardeners. 'Swimmers' shoulder' and 'tennis shoulder' are common in the sporting context, but examples may be found in many situations in which there is repetitive overhead activity.

In the workplace, activities that load the rotator cuff are legion (Figure 4.3). Workers with chronic shoulder–neck complaints (identified by interview or questionnaire) reported significantly more work with their hands at or above shoulder level than control workers (Bjelle *et al.*, 1979). More objective estimates of workload, obtained by filming patients and controls, demonstrated an increase in the duration and frequency of forward flexion or abduction of both arms in cases of acute shoulder pain (Bjelle *et al.*, 1981).

Cleaners and packers have been shown to be at risk on account of frequent rotational movements of the outstretched arms (English *et al.*, 1995). Drivers, miners, construction workers and labourers are other groups in whom rotator cuff disease might be predicted. The prevalence of supraspinatus tendinitis in welders was found to be 18% by Herberts *et al.* (1981). There was no correlation with years spent working and no evidence that rotator cuff tendinitis was an age-dependent phenomenon. By comparison the prevalence in white-collar workers was 2%.

The incidence of rotator cuff tears in cadaveric studies has been reported as between 5% and 32%, although the prevalence of *symptomatic* disease in those cases was unknown (Cofield, 1985).

Both from a medicolegal standpoint (in those cases involving litigation) and from a preventative aspect, the causative factors should be evaluated with some precision in individual cases.

Clinical features

Pain is felt in the C5 dermatome, maximal in the anterolateral aspect of the upper arm, and radiating distally in severe cases to the radial aspect of the forearm and proximally to the base of the neck. In common with frozen shoulder, pain is provoked by lying on the affected side at night. Diurnally, pain is related to activities in which there is repetitive or maintained abduction and/or rotations of the arm(s).

Examination findings

The discerning clinician will note the reproduction of pain (and minor weakness as a result of pain inhibition) on resisted abduction of the arm in supraspinatus tendinitis. By contrast, in subacromial dysfunction that is secondary to cervical spinal joint dysfunction, although active abduction of the shoulder is

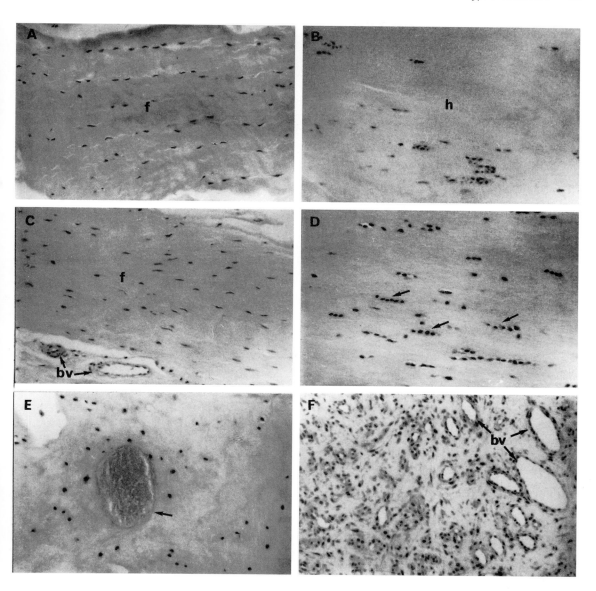

Figure 5.26 Degenerative changes in the human supraspinatus tendon are demonstrated in these specimens (with normal tissue for comparison) prepared by H&E staining. (*A*) 19-year-old cadaver specimen showing normal tendon fibre structure, consisting of organized collagen fibres and parallel aligned tenocytes. (*B*) 88-year-old cadaver specimen showing degenerate tendon with homogenous (hyaline) appearance and regions of acellular matrix. (*C*) 56-year-old patient specimen, showing region of relatively normal tendon with organized collagen fibres with blood vessels in the surrounding loose connective tissue. (*D*) 65-year-old patient specimen, showing region of cell rounding and fibrocartilaginous change (arrows indicate columns of rounded tenocytes). (*E*) 55-year-old patient specimen, showing severely degenerate matrix, with hyaline and hypocellular matrix surrounding a calcific deposit (indicated by arrow). (*F*) 39-year-old patient specimen, showing hypercellular matrix with blood vessel and mononuclear cell infiltration. **f**, normal fibre bundle; **h**, homogenous or hyaline matrix; **bv**, blood vessel; × 107. (Courtesy of Graham Riley, Rheumatology Research Unit, Addenbrooke's Hospital, Cambridge)

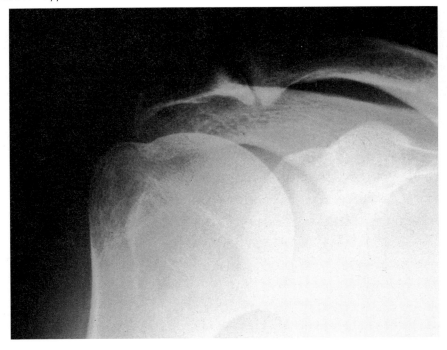

Figure 5.27 Descending osteophytes from the acromioclavicular joint may be a contributory factor in subacromial impingement

demonstrably abnormal – the 'hitch' or arc results from dysco-ordination of the C5/C6 innervated rotator cuff muscles, or possibly from dysco-ordination of the scapular muscles innervated from other spinal levels – there is no pain or specific weakness on resisted contraction of any individual muscle group. In proximal thoracic lesions, patients commonly experience discomfort and difficulty abducting both shoulders simultaneously.

A test of considerable importance is the *impingement sign.* When subacromial impingement is caused by a space-occupying lesion such as an inflamed or torn supraspinatus tendon, the impingement sign is usually positive: internal rotation of the arm, flexed forwards to 90 degrees at the shoulder and flexed to 90 degrees at the elbow, provokes discomfort and is limited in range. The impingement sign is negative (for pain) in neuromuscular disturbances.

If discomfort is experienced when the arm is abducted to 90° and passively externally rotated, anterior *instability* at the glenohumeral joint should be suspected, and excluded by further careful examination (see Chapter 7). Shoulder instability may become symptomatic during (and sometimes caused by) repeated forceful overhead work (Figure 7.17).

Of some importance when active abduction of the arm is painful is the differentiation from adhesive capsulitis of the shoulder, which is one of the few musculoskeletal conditions that is defiantly idiopathic: there is no known relationship with work apart from the subgroup of post-traumatic capsulitis which occurs after an overt injury such as a fall on to the arm or shoulder. All active and passive movements of the glenohumeral joint are restricted in range in adhesive capsulitis: loss of external rotation is the cardinal sign in early lesions. Subsequently, the capsular pattern emerges – greater loss of external rotation than of abduction or internal rotation. Rotator cuff power is retained unless pain inhibition becomes profound. There is no localized tenderness. In my view, it should be treated energetically by intra-articular steroid injections, and subsequently by stretching exercises once the painful inflammatory phase has been overcome.

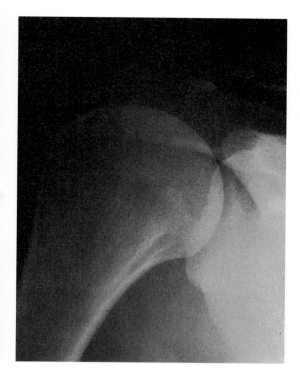

Figure 5.28 Heterotopic calcification in the rotator cuff may contribute to subacromial impingement

The examination findings in subacromial impingement, by contrast, are retention of external rotation, some loss of internal rotation (particularly when combined with forward flexion of the arm in the impingement test), and a painful arc on abduction. Loss of full abduction with terminal pain often indicates a lesion of the acromioclavicular joint. Passive horizontal adduction of the arm is painful and often restricted in range in acromioclavicular strains, whereas it is painless in rotator cuff disease.

Additionally, isometric tests have considerable discriminative value in defining the site of the lesion – most commonly in the supraspinatus tendon, when resisted abduction is painful and/or weak, and less frequently in the other shoulder-stabilizing components of the rotator cuff (infraspinatus and subscapularis).

Palpation may also confirm the site of the rotator cuff lesion. Tenderness is found in cases of tendinitis or partial tear. A defect may be palpated immediately superior to its attachment to the greater tuberosity when the supraspinatus tendon is completely torn (Figure 5.30).

Although the diagnosis of rotator cuff disease is mainly a clinical exercise, further investigations may be useful in selected cases. Radiological abnormalities include ectopic calcification, degenerative changes in the acromioclavicular joint, and elevation of the humeral head (with a chronic rotator cuff tear). MRI is the investigation of choice to demonstrate the extent of supraspinatus tendon pathology (Figure 5.31).

Outcome

Many cases of work-related rotator cuff tendinitis are acute-on-chronic conditions, and respond to conventional treatment modalities. Physiotherapeutic techniques include ice-massage, ultrasound or laser therapy, and rehabilitative exercises once the acute phase has resolved. Medical treatments include non-steroidal anti-inflammatory drugs and rest, but in my experience the most effective strategy is the use of subacromial steroid and local anaesthetic injections for the associated subacromial bursitis (Figure 5.32).

Regrettably, the methodological quality of most studies of the use of steroid injections is poor, and the evidence for the efficacy of steroid injections to the subacromial bursa is scanty. Injected triamcinolone was found by Adebajo *et al.* (1990) to be superior to oral diclofenac (and vastly superior to placebo) in the reduction of pain and improvement in function in patients with rotator cuff tendinitis.

The long-term outcome of rotator cuff tendinitis is far from promising, however (Chard *et al.*, 1988). Twenty-six per cent of patients with rotator cuff tendinitis (diagnosed clinically by positive shoulder pain exacerbation on resisted movements) experienced severe pain after (a mean of) 19 months from presentation. A further 29% were symptomatic to a lesser degree after a similar period of time. All patients received non-surgical treatment, including subacromial steroid injections in most cases. Manual occupation was not related to a worse prognosis, leading the authors to conclude that physical stress was less important than inherent factors such as tendon degeneration. However, those cases associated with overuse from sport or hobbies and those affecting the non-dominant arm

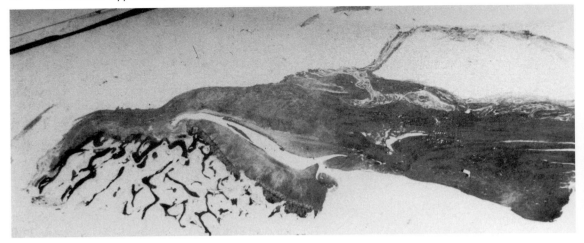

Figure 5.29 A substantial partial tear of the supraspinatus tendon is demonstrated. There is continuity of the superficial fibres. (Courtesy of Professor Hiroaki Fukuda, Tokai University, Japan)

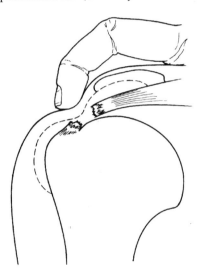

Figure 5.30 The clinical diagnosis of rupture of the supraspinatus tendon is assisted by palpation of the defect. (After E.A. Codman, *The Shoulder: Rupture of the Supraspinatus Tendon*, R.E. Krieger Pub. Co. Inc., Florida, 1934)

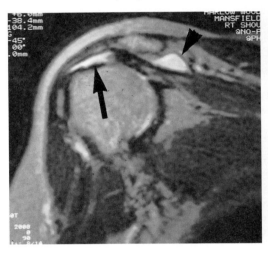

Figure 5.31 MRI is the investigation of choice to demonstrate a supraspinatus tendon tear. On this T2 weighted spin echo oblique coronal image a full thickness tear (*arrow*) of the supraspinatus tendon is demonstrated. The arrow head denotes fluid in the subacromial bursa

fared better, suggesting that reduction in provocative stress leads to more rapid healing.

Lessons for treatment and, particularly, for prevention of occupational shoulder pain may be learnt from sports such as baseball, tennis and front crawl or butterfly swimming in which subacromial impingement secondary to repeated overhead activity is very common (Hutson, 1996). Technical changes, for

instance an alteration in the angle of elevation of the throwing, serving or recovery arm, may be effective in reducing stress on the rotator cuff. Preventative measures to reduce the prevalence of overuse syndromes at the shoulder and elsewhere in the upper limb appear to be more widely practised in the professional arts than in industry.

Both arthroscopic and open acromioplasty have a good success rate in the established

and resection of the acromioclavicular ligament; the non-operative regimen consisted of supervised exercises 'to normalize dysfunctional neuromuscular patterns and to increase the nutrition of the collagen in the rotator cuff'. Both treatments compared favourably with placebo (in the form of simulated laser treatment); the non-surgical regimen was less expensive.

In the presence of a complete tear of the rotator cuff, less than 50% of patients with chronic shoulder pain recover with non-surgical treatment. With surgical treatment, in the form of repair of the tear, possibly combined with acromioplasty, 85% excellent or good results may be expected (Cofield, 1985).

MYOFASCIAL PAIN

Muscle hyperalgesia in the neck, upper back, pectoral girdle and upper limb manifests as tenderness, tender points, hypertonus, or trigger points. The *denotation* depends as much on the skill, inclination and experience of the examiner as on the intensity of the hyperalgesia. The *connotation* is explored in Chapters 2 and 3. In summary, the term myofascial pain syndrome (MPS) implies the presence of one or more trigger points (TPs), areas of increased muscle tension within which are taut bands, and referred phenomena. The concept of the myofascial pain syndrome incorporates trigger points as areas of primary hyperalgesia (whereas the alternative hypothesis is that the very same areas of muscle tenderness and hypertonus are areas of secondary hyperalgesia).

Pain and muscle tenderness in the base of the neck or in the adjacent scapular region are commonly found in keyboard operators and machinists, when they are usually associated with sustained contraction of the scalene muscles and/or the proximal scapular fixator muscles (upper trapezius, levator scapulae and rhomboids). The referred pain pattern from stimulation of the trigger points in the scaleni includes the pectoral region, the medial scapular region and the radial aspect of the arm as far as the radial digits (Figure 3.11). The levator scapulae trigger point refers pain to the back of the shoulder and to the medial border of the scapula, though the most

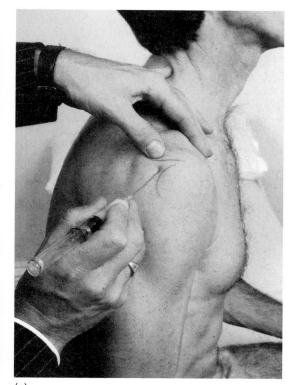

(a)

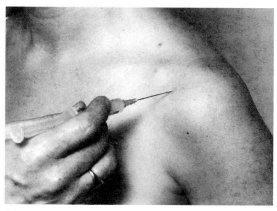

(b)

Figure 5.32 Subacromial steroid injections are often effective in subacromial impingement: (*a*) the posterior approach; (*b*) the anterior approach

impingement syndrome. When comparing surgery and a supervised exercise regimen for stage 2 rotator cuff lesions, Brox found equally good improvement after both. Surgery consisted of bursectomy, partial acromionectomy

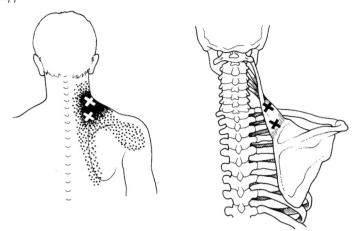

Figure 5.33 The trigger points and pain reference zones from the levator scapulae muscle. (After Travell and Simons, 1983)

intense pain is felt locally (Travell and Simons, 1983) (Figure 5.33).

As muscle hypertonus in the proximal scapular fixators – adjacent to the superomedial angle of the scapula – is so common, its significance depends on the presence of additional examination findings. As a form of secondary hyperalgesia, it may be associated with spinal joint dysfunction in the distal cervical or upper thoracic spine, from which primary myofascial pain must be differentiated. In general, its common associates are whiplash injuries to the neck, occupations in which the arms are frequently held unsupported in front of the body, cervical disc prolapse and neuropathic arm pain.

It is unusual for workers to be so disabled as to lose time from work as a result of scapular pain; the symptoms in some occupations are almost endemic. The two situations in which posterior shoulder pain of this type becomes more intrusive are:

(a) when there is an underlying cervicodorsal spinal joint dysfunction or intervertebral disc prolapse (in which case there are likely to be referred symptoms through the arm in a radicular or segmental pattern and typical articular signs on examining the cervical spine);

(b) when there are features of neuropathic arm pain – in which there is widespread hyperalgesia throughout the limb.

CERVICAL SPINAL LESIONS

Pathoanatomy and pathophysiology

It is universally accepted that radicular symptoms in the arm usually indicate nerve root entrapment secondary to a paracentral disc protrusion or, in the older population, to foraminal bony hypertrophy (Figure 3.6). Nerve root pain may be very distressing, and is often incompatible with manual or office work for a variable period of time, depending upon the pathology.

By contrast, the orthodox medical profession has experienced difficulty in recognizing the concept of cervical spinal joint dysfunction and, as a corollary, its role in certain types of WRULD. This is hardly surprising as the diagnosis and management of functional disorders of the spine continue to be poorly understood outwith the disciplines of musculoskeletal or osteopathic medicine. As yet, dysfunctional conditions of the spine (often referred to as benign 'mechanical' spinal conditions) attract little attention from the major disciplines of orthopaedics and rheumatology.

Epistemological enlightenment would lead to a more widespread rejection by clinicians of the completely discredited association between the (radiological) condition of cervical spondylosis – indicating age-related changes in the cervical spine – and neck and arm pain. Such an archaic view regarding a proposed association between symptoms and radiographic findings promotes arbitrariness of diagnosis and indifference to aetiology. Age-related degenerative changes develop inexorably in the general population – they are present in 90% of 65-year-olds (Lawrence, 1969) – but there is poor correlation with symptoms.

Equally devastating epistemologically is the medical 'comfort zone' created by 'positive' MRI findings of disc prolapse and nerve root entrapment or displacement to explain refractory neck and arm pain. As yet there are no longitudinal studies correlating the less spectacular MRI changes of disc degeneration/disc bulging with neck and arm pain. Nevertheless, pathological changes of disc degeneration, indicating loss of shock-absorption, and in more severe cases disc 'failure', offer a more realistic basis for an association between spinal pain and referred pain to the arm in some cases.

A helpful concept is that of segmental *spinal joint (somatic) dysfunction* based upon a neural (reflex) pathogenesis – and affected by posture, environmental stresses and adverse biomechanics. Reversible spinal joint dysfunction is a clinical diagnosis with characteristic features that reflect the severity of the condition. The following syndromes are recognized.

1   Localized neck pain (somatic dysfunction with a localized zone of irritation).
2   Localized neck pain and referred pain (somatic dysfunction with both localized and peripheral zones of irritation).
3   Neck and widespread persistent arm pain (somatic dysfunction as in (2) above but with neural sensitization).

Aetiology

Although neck pain may exist without pain referred to the arm, this is not usually classified as a WRULD. Nevertheless, posture at work may play an important aetiological role in the onset and/or aggravation of neck pain. Clearly, disturbances of the cervical spine for whatever reason – pathoanatomical or pathoneurophysiological – are commonly associated with arm pain. From the aspect of causation, the temporal and dose–response relationships between cervical spinal dysfunction and occupation should be explored in individual patients.

Clinical features

The symptomatology is dependent upon the segmental level of dysfunction and its severity. It is convenient to differentiate between proximal cervical, mid-cervical and cervicodorsal lesions. For convenience, the upper thoracic spine will be included in the latter category.

Proximal

Dovey (1989) states that the apparently dissociated clinical features arising from dysfunction at C0–1 and C1–2 can only be explained on the basis of the proximity of the proximal spinal joints to the cranial nerve nuclei in the brain stem. Occipital headache, radiating to the frontal region, is common. Less frequent, but well recognized, are disturbances of balance (vertigo), disturbances of hearing (tinnitus) and disturbances of vision (diplopia, nystagmus). Feelings of disorientation, depression and lack of concentration are common complaints of patients with proximal cervical lesions after whiplash (and equally commonly diagnosed – often inappropriately – as post-traumatic stress or post-concussive states) but are less frequently encountered as occupational disorders. Lesions at C2–3 often give maxillofacial pain.

Mid-cervical

Mid-cervical lesions are characterized by unilateral neck pain, radiating to the scapular region. Peripheral zones of irritation (which are not always symptomatic) may be detectable as tender points. Smythe (1994) describes tender points in the C5–6 syndrome at the mid-trapezius, supraspinatus origin, lateral elbow and second costochondral junction. In the C6–7 syndrome the tender points are the origin and insertion of pectoralis minor (coracoid tip and fourth/fifth ribs in the lateral chest wall), interscapular region and medial elbow (Figure 5.34). Scapular pain is a particularly common and often distressing feature to the patient. Referred pain and dysaesthesiae may be present throughout the arm and hand; by contrast, if there is nerve root compression at either of these described levels, the radicular symptoms of pain, numbness and

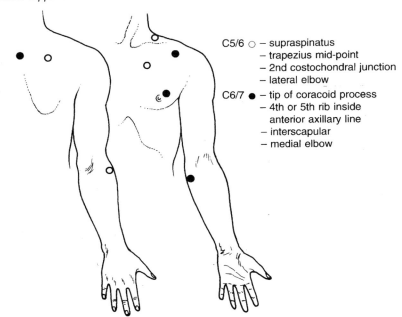

C5/6 ○ – supraspinatus
– trapezius mid-point
– 2nd costochondral junction
– lateral elbow
C6/7 ● – tip of coracoid process
– 4th or 5th rib inside
 anterior axillary line
– interscapular
– medial elbow

Figure 5.34 Tender points in characteristic sites have been described by Smythe (1994) in the C5–6 and C6–7 syndromes

paraesthesiae have a much more defined segmental – dermatomal – pattern.

Cervicodorsal

Pain is usually felt in the midline at the cervicodorsal junctional region or paravertebrally in the proximal interscapular region. A small (axial) area of hypoaesthesia is not uncommon. Discomfort and dysaesthesiae often radiate to the arm, particularly along the ulnar border. Spasm of the medial scapular muscles is a marked feature.

The cervical spinal movements are of full range and pain-free other than extension, which is usually painful when lesions are centred upon C7 or D1. Active abduction of both shoulders is restricted when the dysfunction affects the upper thoracic spine. Vasomotor changes, including oedema of the hand, may be present (Fraser, 1990).

Examination findings
Nerve root entrapment secondary to a cervical intervertebral disc prolapse usually gives rise to the articular pattern described by Cyriax: some active movements are painful, others not. Rotation to the painful side is nearly always painful, and often restricted with a twingey end-feel. The combination of extension and ipsilateral rotation often reproduces the arm pain and paraesthesiae. Tenderness of the anterolateral margin of the C5–6 or C6–7 disc may be detected.

Positive neurological signs, particularly motor weakness, confirm the level of root paresis. When the articular signs are relatively minor, or absent, and there are no abnormal neurological signs in the upper limb, tests for abnormal neural tension should be used (see Chapter 7).

In cervical spinal joint dysfunction there is a variable degree of painful limitation of cervical movements. Segmental signs include spinous process tenderness, paravertebral muscle hypertonus and loss of joint play (accessory movements). Fixation of the first rib (an osteopathic concept indicating loss of movement with respiration) is sometimes found with cervicodorsal junctional lesions. In upper thoracic spinal joint dysfunction, discomfort on neck extension, loss of full abduction of the shoulders and segmental compression discomfort are the principal features.

The location of secondary muscle hyperalgesia is related to the segmental level of dysfunction, as already described. Muscle tenderness along the medial border of the scapula is a common examination finding, particularly as the examiner's attention is drawn to this region by the patient's symptoms. However, other tender points in the upper limb may be palpated during a careful examination.

Conclusion

Historically the relationship between diffuse pains around the shoulder girdle and cervical lesions has been recognized (Cyriax, 1969). More recently, distinct patterns of 'tender points' or 'trigger points' in the neck, shoulder girdle and upper limb have been demonstrated with cervical spinal syndromes (Smythe, 1988, 1994).

The need for a detailed history and a comprehensive musculoskeletal examination that includes the cervicodorsal spine is paramount in the assessment of all upper limb disorders. The function of the cervical spine at each segmental level should be carefully assessed, and the presence and extent of muscle hyperalgesia (tender points, trigger points) in the neck, upper back, shoulders and arms should be established.

As described in Chapter 6, cervicodorsal spinal lesions may be implicated in the pathogenesis of type 2 WRULD, in which neural or soft tissue injury, axial or peripheral, is thought to be the cause of pathological sensorineural processing within the central nervous system, inducing the development of widespread hyperalgesia, extending from the neck into the affected limb. Widespread TPs with right–left and upper body–lower body symmetry suggest fibromyalgia.

References

Adebajo, A.O., Nash, P. and Hazleman, B.L. (1990) A prospective double blind dummy placebo controlled study comparing triamcinolone with oral diclofenac 50 mg tds in patients with rotator cuff tendinitis. *J. Rheumatol.*, **17**, 1207–10.

Bejjani, F.J., Kaye, G.M. and Benham, M. (1996) Musculoskeletal and neuromuscular conditions of instrumental musicians. *Arch. Phys. Med. Rehabil.*, **77**, 406–13.

Bianchi, L. (1878) A contribution on the treatment of the professional dyscinesiae. *Br. Med. J.*, **1**, 87–9.

Bjelle, A., Hagberg, M. and Michaelsson, G. (1979) Clinical and ergonomic factors in prolonged shoulder pain among industrial workers. *Scand. J. Work Environ. Health*, **5**, 205–10.

Bjelle, A., Hagberg, M. and Michaelsson, G. (1981) Occupational and individual factors in acute shoulder–neck disorders among industrial workers. *Br. J. Ind. Med.*, **38**, 356–63.

Bonnici, A.V. and Spencer, J.D. (1988) A survey of trigger finger in adults. *J. Hand Surg.*, **13B**, 202–3.

Boyd, H.B. and McLeod, A.C. (1973) Tennis elbow. *J. Bone Joint Surg.*, **55A**(6), 1183–7.

Braidwood, A.S. (1975) Superficial radial neuropathy. *J. Bone Joint Surg.*, **57B**, 380–3.

Brain, W.R., Wright, A.D. and Wilkinson, M. (1947) Spontaneous compression of both median nerves in the carpal tunnel: six cases treated surgically. *Lancet*, **1**, 277–82.

Braun, R.M., Davidson, K. and Doehr, S. (1989) Provocative testing in the diagnosis of dynamic carpal tunnel syndrome. *J. Hand Surg.*, **14A**, 195–7.

Brox, J.I., Staff, P.H., Ljunggren, A.E. and Brevik, J.I. (1993) Arthroscopic surgery compared with supervised exercises in patients with rotator cuff disease (stage 2 impingement syndrome). *Br. Med. J.*, **307**, 899–903.

Cawston, T.R., Riley, G.P. and Hazleman, B.L. (1996) Tendon lesions and soft tissue rheumatism – great outback or great opportunity? *Ann. Rheum. Dis.*, **55**, 1–3.

Chard, M.D. and Hazleman, B.L. (1989) Tennis elbow – a reappraisal. *Br. J. Rheumatol.*, **28**(3), 186–8.

Chard, M.D., Sattelle, L.M. and Hazleman, B.L. (1988) The long-term outcome of rotator cuff tendinitis – a review study. *Br. J. Rheumatol.*, **27**, 385–9.

Cofield, R.H. (1985) Rotator cuff disease of the shoulder. *J. Bone Joint Surg.*, **67A**(6), 974–9.

Cohen, L., Hallett, M., Geller, B. *et al.* (1987) Treatment of focal dystonias of the hand with botulinum toxin injection. *Neurology*, **37**, Suppl. 1, 123–4.

Coonrad, R.W. and Hooper, W.R. (1973) Tennis elbow: its course, natural history, conservative and surgical management. *J. Bone Joint Surg.*, **55A**, 1177.

Cyriax, J.H. (1936) The pathology and treatment of tennis elbow. *J. Bone Joint Surg.*, **18**, 921–40.

Cyriax, J.H. (1969) *Textbook of Orthopaedic Medicine: Diagnosis of Soft-tissue Lesions*, 5th edn. Baillière, Tindall, Cassell, London, p. 337.

Dovey, H. (1989) The cervical spine and brachial neuralgia. *J. Orthop. Med.*, **11**(3), 61–4.

Dums, F. (1896) Uber trommlerlahmungen. *Deutsch. Militarztliche Zeitschr.*, **25**, 144–55.

Dupuytren, Baron G. (1834) Permanent retraction of the fingers, produced by an affection of the palmar fascia. *Lancet*, **ii**, 222–5.

English, C.J., MacLaren, W.M., Court-Brown, C., Hughes, S.P.F. *et al.* (1995) Relations between upper limb soft tissue disorders and repetitive movements at work. *Am. J. Industr. Med.*, **27**(1), 75–90.

Evans, J.A. (1947) Reflex sympathetic dystrophy. *Ann. Intern. Med.*, **26**, 417–26.

Feldman, R.G., Travers, P.H., Chirico-Post, J. and Keyserling, W.M. (1987) Risk assessment in electronic assembly workers: carpal tunnel syndrome. *J. Hand Surg.*, **12A**(5), 849–55.

Foster, R.J. and Edshage, S. (1981) Factors related to the outcome of surgically managed compressive ulnar neuropathy at the elbow level. *J. Hand Surg.*, **6**(2), 181–92.

Fraser, D.M. (1990) T3 syndrome. In: *Back Pain – an International Review*, (eds J.K. Paterson and L. Burn), Kluwer Academic, Lancaster.

Gelberman, R.H., Rydevik, B.L., Pess, G.M., Szabo, R.M. and Lundborg, G. (1988) Carpal tunnel syndrome. *Orthop. Clin. North Am.*, **19**(1), 115–24.

Gellman, H. (1992) Tennis elbow (lateral epicondylitis). *Orthop. Clin. North Am.*, **23**(1), 75–82.

Goldie, I. (1964) Epicondylitis lateralis humeri (epicondylalgia or tennis elbow): a pathologic study. *Acta Chir. Scand. Suppl.*, 339.

Golding, D.N. (1986) Tennis and golfer's elbow. *Reports on Rheumatic Diseases*, 2. Arthritis and Rheumatism Council, London.

Gowers, W.R. (1883) *A Manual of Diseases of the Nervous System*, 2nd edn. Reprinted by Hafner Publishing Co., Darien, CT, 1970.

Gruchow, H.W. and Pelletier, B.S. (1979) An epidemiologic study of tennis elbow. *Am. J. Sports Med.*, **7**, 234–8.

Hadler, N.M. (1993) *Occupational Musculoskeletal Disorders*. Raven Press, New York, pp. 198–9.

Harvey, F.J., Harvey, P.M. and Horsley, M.W. (1990) de Quervain's disease: surgical or non-surgical treatment. *J. Hand Surg.*, **15A**, 83–7.

Herberts, P., Kadefors, R., Andersson, G. and Petersen, I. (1981) Shoulder pain in industry: an epidemiological study on welders. *Acta Orthop. Scand.*, **52**, 299–306.

Herrick, A.L. (1994) Reflex sympathetic dystrophy. *Reports on Rheumatic Diseases*, 2. Arthritis and Rheumatism Council, London.

Hochberg, F.H., Leffert, R.D. and Heler, M.D. (1983) Hand difficulties among musicians. *JAMA*, **249**, 1869–72.

Hooper, G. and McMaster, M.J. (1979) Stenosing tenovaginitis affecting the tendon of extensor digiti minimi at the wrist. *Hand*, **11**, 29–301.

Howard F.M. (1986) Controversies in nerve entrapment syndromes in the forearm and wrist. *Orthop. Clin. North Am.*, **17**(3), 375–81.

Hutson, M.A. (1996) *Sports Injuries: Recognition and Management*, 2nd edn. Oxford University Press, Oxford.

Ireland, D.C.R. (1988) Psychological and physical aspects of occupational arm pain. *J. Bone Jt. Surg.*, **13B**(1), 5–10.

Industrial Injuries Advisory Council (1992) *Work Related Upper Limb Disorders*. HMSO, London.

Janig, W. (1990) The sympathetic nervous system in pain: physiology and pathophysiology. In: *Pain and the Sympathetic Nervous System* (ed. M. Stanton-Hicks), Kluwer Academic, Mass., pp. 17–89.

Katz, J.N., Larson, M.G., Sabra, A. *et al.* (1990) The carpal tunnel syndrome: diagnostic utility of the history and physical examination findings. *Ann. Intern. Med.*, **112**, 321–7

Keenan, J. (1991) Carpal tunnel syndrome: a personal view of a common problem. *J. Orthop. Med.*, **13**(2), 43–5.

Kiefhaber, T.R. and Stern, P.J. (1992) Upper extremity tendinitis and overuse syndromes in the athlete. *Clin. Sports Med.*, **11**(1), 39–55.

Kivi, P. (1982) The aetiology and conservative treatment of humeral epicondylitis. *Scand. J. Rehabil. Med.*, **15**, 37–41.

Kopell, H.P. and Thompson, W.A.L. (1963). *Peripheral Entrapment Neuropathies*. Williams & Wilkins, Baltimore, Md.

Koskimies, K., Farkkila, M., Pyykko, J., Jantti, V. *et al.* (1990) Carpal tunnel syndrome in vibration disease. *Br. J. Industr. Med.*, **47**, 411–16.

Kuchera, M.L. (1995) Gravitational stress, musculoligamentous strain, and postural alignment. *Spine State Art Rev.*, **9**(2), 463–90.

Kurppa, K., Waris, P. and Rokkanen, P. (1979) Tennis elbow, lateral elbow pain syndrome. *Scand. J. Work Environ. Health*, **5** (Suppl. 3), 15–18.

Kuschner, S.H., Ebramzadeh, E., Johnson, D., Brien, W.W. and Sherman, R. (1992) Tinel's sign and Phalen's test in carpal tunnel syndrome. *Orthopaedics*, **15**, 1297–1302.

Lapidus, P.W. and Guidotti, F.P. (1972) Stenosing tenovaginitis of the wrist and fingers. *Clin. Orthop.*, **83**, 87–90.

Lawrence, J.S. (1969) Disc degeneration: its frequency and relation to symptoms. *Ann. Rheum. Dis.*, **28**, 121–38.

Leao, L. (1958) de Quervain's disease: a clinical and anatomical study. *J. Bone Joint Surg.*, **40A**(5), 1063–70.

Lederman, R.J. (1988) Occupational cramp in instrumental musicians. *Med. Prob. Performing Artists*, **3**(2), 45–51.

Lederman, R.J. (1991). Focal dystonia in instrumentalists: clinical features. *Med. Prob. Performing Artists*, 6(4), 132–6.

Lundborg, G., Sollerman, C., Stromberg, T. and Pyykko, J. (1987) A new principle for assessment of vibrotactile sense in vibration-induced neuropathy. *Scand. J. Work Environ. Health*, **13**, 375–9.

Major, H.P. (1883) Lawn-tennis elbow. *Br. Med. J.*, **ii**, 557.

Marks, M.R. and Gunther, S.F. (1989) Efficacy of cortisone treatment in treatment of trigger fingers and thumbs. *J. Hand Surg.*, **14A**, 722–7.

Masear, V.R., Hayes, J.M. and Hyde, A.G. (1986) An industrial cause of carpal tunnel syndrome. *J. Hand Surg.*, **11A**, 222–7.

Mills, G.P. (1928) The treatment of tennis elbow. *Br. Med. J.*, **1**, 12–13.

Mills, K.R. (1985) Orthodromic sensory action potentials from palmar stimulation in the diagnosis of carpal tunnel syndrome. *J. Neurol. Neurosurg. Psychiat.*, **48**, 250–5.

Morris, H. (1882) Rider's sprain. *Lancet*, **ii**, 557.

Mossman, S.S. and Blau, J.N. (1989) Tinel's sign and the carpal tunnel syndrome. *J. Orthop. Med.*, **11**(3), 72.

Nathan, P.A., Meadows, K.D. and Doyle, L.S. (1988) Occupation as a risk factor for impaired sensory conduction of the median nerve at the carpal tunnel. *J. Hand Surg.*, **13B**, 167–70.

Nelson, C.L., Sawmiller, S. and Phalen, G.S. (1972) Ganglions of the wrist and hand. *J. Bone Joint Surg.*, **54A**, 1459–64.

Newmark, J. and Hochberg, F.H. (1987) Isolated painless manual incoordination in fifty-seven musicians. *J. Neurol, Neurosurg. Psychiat.*, **50**, 291–5.

Niepel, G.A. and Sit'aj, S. (1979) Enthesopathy. *Clin. Rheumatol. Dis.*, **5**(3), 857–72.

Nirschl, R.P. (1986) Soft-tissue injuries about the elbow. *Clin. Sports Med.*, **5**(4), 637–52.

Nirschl, R.P. and Pettrone, F.A. (1979) The surgical treatment of lateral epicondylitis. *J. Bone Joint Surg.*, **61A**(6), 832–9.

Noble, J., Arafa, M., Royle, S.G., McGeorge, G. and Crank, S. (1992) The association between alcohol, hepatic pathology and Dupuytren's disease. *J. Hand Surg.*, **17B**, 71–4.

Oppenheim, H. (1911) *Textbook of Nervous Diseases*, 5th edn., T.N. Foulis, London.

Pellegrini, V.D. (1992) Osteoarthritis at the base of the thumb. *Orthop. Clin. North Am.*, **23**(1), 83–102.

Pfeffer, G.B., Gelberman, R.H., Boyes, J.H. and Rydevik, B. (1988) The history of carpal tunnel syndrome. *J. Hand Surg.*, **13B**(1), 28–34.

Phalen, G.S. (1966) The carpal-tunnel syndrome – seventeen years' experience in diagnosis and treatment of six hundred and fifty-four hands. *J. Bone Joint Surg.*, **48A**, 211–28.

Phalen, G.S. (1972) The carpal-tunnel syndrome. *Clin. Orthop. Rel. Res.*, **83**, 29–40.

Phalen, G.S., Gardner, W.J. and Lalonde, A.A. (1950) Neuropathy of the median nerve due to compression beneath the transverse carpal ligament. *J. Bone Joint Surg.*, **32A**(1), 109–12.

Plewes, L.W. (1956) Sudeck's atrophy in the hand. *J. Bone Joint Surg.*, **38B**, 195–203.

Poore, G.V. (1887) Clinical lecture on certain conditions of the hand and arm which interfere with the performance of professional acts, especially piano-playing. *Br. Med. J.*, **1**, 441–4.

de Quervain F. (1895) Ueber eine form von chronischer tendovaginitis. (Correspondenz – Blatt F.) *Schweizer Arzte*, **25**, 389–94.

Quinnell, R.C. (1980) Conservative management of trigger finger. *Practitioner*, **224**, 187–90.

Ramazzini, B. (1713) *De morbis artificum diatriba.* Padua. (Trans. W.C. Wright (1940) in *Diseases of Workers*, Hafner Publishing Co. Inc., New York.)

Rathbun, J.B. and MacNab, I. (1970) The microvascular pattern of the rotator cuff. *J. Bone Joint Surg.*, **52B**, 540–53.

Renton, J. (1830) Observations on acupuncture. *Edinb. Med. Surg. J.*, **34**, 100–107.

Rhoades, C.E., Gelberman, R.H. and Manjarris, J.F. (1984) Stenosing tenosynovitis of the fingers and thumb. *Clin. Orthop. Rel. Res.*, **190**, 236–8.

Roles, N.C. and Maudsley, R.H. (1972) Radial tunnel syndrome: resistant tennis elbow as a nerve entrapment. *J. Bone Joint Surg.*, **54B**(3), 499–508.

Romberg, M.H. (1853) *A Manual of the Nervous Diseases of Man*, vol. 1 (trans. E.H. Sieveking). Sydenham Society, London, pp. 320–4.

Rosenbaum, R.B. and Ochoa, J.L. (1993) *Carpal Tunnel Syndrome and Other Disorders of the Median Nerve.* Butterworth–Heinemann, Stoneham, Mass., pp. 233–49.

Runge, F. (1873) Zur genese und behandlung des schreibekrampfes. *Berl. Klin. Wochensch.*, **10**, 245–8.

Semple, J.C. and Cargill, A.O. (1969) Carpal-tunnel syndrome. Results of surgical decompression. *Lancet*, **1**, 918–19.

Silverstein, B.A., Fine, L.J., Armstrong, T.J. (1987) Occupational factors and carpal tunnel syndrome. *Am. J. Ind. Med.*, **11**, 343–58.

Smith, E.M., Sonstegard, D.A. and Anderson, W.H. (1977) Carpal tunnel syndrome: contribution of flexor tendons. *Arch. Phys. Med. Rehabil.*, **58**, 379–85.

Smythe, H.A. (1988) The 'repetitive strain injury syndrome' is referred pain from the neck. *J. Rheumatol.*, **15**(11), 1604–8.

Smythe, H.A. (1994) The C6–7 syndrome – clinical features and treatment response. *J. Rheumatol.*, **21**(8), 1520–26.

Spinner, M. (1970) The anterior interosseous nerve syndrome. *J. Bone Joint Surg.*, **52A**(1), 84–94.

Spinner, M. and Olshansky, K. (1973) The extensor indicis proprius syndrome: a clinical test. *Plast. Reconstr. Surg.*, **51**(2), 134–8.

Szabo, R.M. and Madison, M. (1992) Carpal tunnel syndrome. *Orthop. Clin. North Am.*, **23**(1), 103–9.

Thompson, A.R., Plewes, L.W. and Shaw, E.G. (1951) Peritendinitis crepitans and simple tenosynovitis: a clinical study of 544 cases in industry. *Br. J. Industr. Med.*, **8**, 150–8.

Thorson, E. and Szabo, R.M. (1992) Common tendinitis problems in the hand and forearm. *Orthop. Clin. North Am.*, **23**(1), 65–74.

Tillaux, P. (1892) *Traité d'anatomie topographique. Avec applications à la chirugie*, Ed. 7. Asselin et Houzeau, Paris.

Travell, J.G. and Simons, D.G. (1983). *The Trigger Point Manual*. Williams & Wilkins, Baltimore, Md.

Troell, A. (1918) Uber die sogenannte tendovaginitis crepitans. *Dtsch., Z. Chir.*, **143**, 125–62.

Upton, A.R.M. and McComas, A.J. (1973) The double crush in nerve-entrapment syndromes. *Lancet*, **ii**, 359–62.

Velpeau, A. (1841) *Crepitation douloureuse des tendons*. Article 2; *Leçons orales de clinique chirurgicale a l'Hôpital de la Charité*, vol. 3, 94, Gernser-Baillière, Paris.

Wadsworth, T.G. (1987) Tennis elbow: conservative, surgical, and manipulative treatment. *Br. Med. J.*, **294**, 621–4.

Wartenberg, R. (1932). Cheiralgia paraesthetica. *Zeitschr. Neurol. Psychiat.*, **141**, 145–55.

Wieslander, G., Norback, D., Gothe, C-J. and Juhlin, L. (1989) Carpal tunnel syndrome and exposure to vibration, repetitive wrist movements, and heavy manual work: a case referent study. *Br. J. Industr. Med.*, **46**, 43–7.

Winckworth, C.E. (1883) Lawn-tennis elbow. *Br. Med. J.*, **ii**, 708.

6

Type 2 WRULDs

No one can doubt that the syndrome will shortly be conscripted into the swelling ranks of so-called psycho-neurotic disorders from which it will, with difficulty, be rescued for medicine proper.

Sir Francis Walshe (1945)

The diffuse form of work-related upper limb disorder (type 2 WRULD), a regional pain syndrome, is characterized by widespread pain and dysaesthesiae in the upper limb. It differs from the specific entities that are categorized as type 1 WRULD in that sufferers from the type 2 disorder experience symptoms that are disseminated throughout the upper limb, neck, shoulder girdles and upper back, and which persist in the established case for prolonged periods of time despite rest. It has frequently been described as a diffuse condition with no evidence of musculoskeletal 'disease' and no objective signs of abnormality – but this is not a correct assessment (see below, Examination findings).

Pathogenesis

A more appropriate term for type 2 WRULD that reflects its pathogenesis is **neuropathic arm pain (NAP)**. As explained in Chapter 3, neurosensitization has two components: peripheral and central. The initial trigger to both components is soft tissue injury or inflammation in the neck or arms, causing stimulation of nociceptive unmyelinated primary afferents. The form of soft tissue injury is either somatic disturbance (for instance apophyseal joint strain, tendon microtrauma or muscle fatigue) or neural dysfunction. If neural, the site may be axial (the cervical spine, or possibly the cervicodorsal junction) or peripheral (for instance peripheral nerve irritation).

In susceptible individuals the barrage of nociceptive input into the spinal cord results in central sensitization in which there is increased excitability of wide dynamic range (WDR) neurones in the dorsal horn. This central hyperexcitability is maintained by neurotransmitters, released from nociceptive C and A fibres, increasing N-methyl-D-aspartate (NMDA) receptor activation. The neuropeptide substance P enhances the activity of NMDA receptors (Kidd *et al.*, 1996).

The dorsal horn neurones are influenced by descending neuronal activity from the higher centres of the central nervous system, by the autonomic nervous system, and by peripheral afferent activity. The normal sensorineural mechanisms for pain production and perception are augmented by the sensitization of the WDR neurones, resulting in *pain amplification* via the additional perception of pain from normally non-painful stimulation of low threshold mechanoreceptors. Thus, central sensitization is characterized by allodynia (reduced thresholds), hyperalgesia (increased response to afferent input), wind-up (increased response to repeated stimulation), hyperpathia (prolonged response to afferent stimulation) and the expansion of receptive fields.

To date, there have been few clinical studies of neuropathia in patients with refractory upper limb pain. However, reduction in pain tolerance, associated with spread of sensation and sustained dysaesthesiae in the upper limb following electrocutaneous electrical stimulation (using a TENS machine) was reported in patients with type 2 WRULD by Arroyo and Cohen (1992). They concluded that the limbs were essentially regions of *secondary hyperaesthesia*. The involvement of the autonomic nervous system in keyboard operators with chronic forearm pain in whom specific conditions were excluded was suggested by the detection of computer assisted thermographic changes (Sharma *et al.*, 1997).

Vulnerability

Although the pathophysiology is becoming clearer, the reason for the activation of neurosensitization in the vulnerable patient is unknown. It is widely suspected that psychological factors play an important role, leading to the concept of psychological vulnerability. Many observers (for instance Pell, 1994) have noted that depressive neurosis is common in those patients with type 2 WRULD. Many of these patients, most frequently females, are conscientious workers, working long hours, and with a long history of stress-associated complaints such as headaches, irritable bowel, depression and anxiety. Difficulties with personal relationships and work stress are common. Another group of patients have minimal intrinsic stress factors, but are subjected to severe extrinsic stressors such as divorce or financial hardship. In these groups muscle tension is common and is often associated with suboccipital and proximal scapular myofascial trigger points.

Assessment of the relationship between psychological vulnerability and neck and arm pain is far from straightforward, however. Few epidemiological studies have attempted to identify the various components of the psychological reaction (such as personality vulnerability, workplace stress, or attitude to disability) and how these components interact with biological and ergonomic factors to produce the final picture (McDermott, 1986). Acknowledging that musculoskeletal symptoms and stress-linked complaints are commonly associated, the question of whether the reporting of both is contingent upon an overall negative attitude to working life was addressed by Pheasant (1992). He concluded that the psychogenic element of the type 2 WRULD syndrome stems principally from the exogenous stresses of working life rather than from an intrinsic psychological vulnerability.

The recognition of abnormal behavioural responses to previous illnesses or injuries is a further factor to consider, and one that is likely to have a significant bearing on the prognosis of the upper limb disorder.

Aetiology

Whatever the pathogenesis of work-related upper limb disorders, whether type 1 or type 2, it is sound clinical practice to identify the stressors in each individual case. In susceptible people neuromuscular, ergonomic and psychogenic factors may all contribute. Prolonged static muscle tension and work stress (in particular) are presumed by many observers to play an important role in the development of the *early* stage of type 2 WRULD.

Studies on work activities suggest that reduction in intramuscular blood flow is the primary cause of muscle fatigue in static loading. Intramuscular circulation is impaired when isometric contraction approaches 20% of maximum contraction. Capillary occlusion results in tissue ischaemia and delayed clearance of metabolites (Karlsson and Ollander, 1972). Repetitive or sustained elevation of the arms at shoulder height and above is a recognized strain upon the rotator cuff (see Figure 4.3). Blanching during arm abduction has been demonstrated by Rathbun and McNab (1970), suggesting that reduced vascularization is a probable factor in rotator cuff degeneration. The frequent use of the pinch grip is stressful; as much as four to five times the normal muscle force is exerted than in the power grip (Armstrong and Chaffin, 1979).

It has been postulated that the pain generated from sustained muscle contraction results from anaerobic metabolism with the accumulation of acids (such as lactic acid and pyruvic acid) and the production of neurotransmitters. Nociceptive pain fibres are stimulated (Helme *et al.*, 1990) leading to the possibility of reflex, sustained muscle spasm and a subsequent vicious cycle of further pain and spasm. This may account for the endemic, if low-grade, discomfort in the neck and shoulders in many workers in light industry, such as sewing machinists (see Figure 4.4), and discomfort in the hands, wrists and forearms in keyboard (and computer mouse) operators.

With respect to ergonomics, an association between demanding manual work and the development of symptoms is sought. Causation may be far from clear-cut however, as the increase (or alteration) in physical stress, following which a compensated biological state is converted to an uncompensated state, may be subtle or relatively minor. This is comparable to the situation with those sports injuries that result from overuse or overload. In general, a change of working practice is often found. In common with type 1 WRULDs, symptoms may arise after a period of rest from work, such as a vacation or pregnancy. Revised management demands, leading to a change of equipment, a change of work-station, a change of work-station layout or a change of manual tasks, are also common stressors. A history of intense work pressure, including working through lunch or rest periods, or working overtime for instance, is a frequent admission by patients at interview.

A dose–response relationship and a temporal relationship between symptoms and work activity should be identifiable in the early stages of type 2 WRULD, but the established case is characterized by 'constant' pain, dysaesthesiae and disability.

Epidemiology

The paucity of meaningful epidemiological studies bedevils the whole spectrum of work-related upper limb disorders. This is true for type 2 as for the discrete conditions within the type 1 category. There is little information on the frequency of type 2 WRULD in the general population and, regrettably, there are few studies in which comparisons are made with control groups of subjects. In most studies, type 2 WRULD is not differentiated from type 1 conditions.

In most studies females are stated to be affected more frequently than males. Cohen *et al.* (1992) stated that in his large series of patients 'with disorders from the severe end of the spectrum (by virtue of the referral process)' the condition arose predominantly in women aged between 20 and 50 years. Office employees (principally keyboard operatives) and manual process workers comprise the majority of his cases. It is not always clear from the majority of studies whether the predominance of females simply reflects the gender ratio in the relevant workforce or whether there is a true increased incidence in females.

In Japan the complaints of neck and arm pain, labelled occupational cervicobrachial disorder (OCD), became sufficiently widespread amongst punch-card perforators, typists, telephone operators, office keyboard operators and assembly line workers in the 1960s and the 1970s for the Japanese Association of Industrial Health to establish a special investigative group. OCD was defined as a 'functional and/or organic disturbance that resulted from neuromuscular fatigue due to work in a fixed position and/or to repetitive movement of the upper extremities' (McDermott, 1986). It would appear that the term OCD encompassed both type 1 and type 2 upper limb disorders.

Against this background of musculoskeletal complaints, Ohara (1976) conducted a comparative study of Japanese female cash register operators, office machine operators and other office workers (mainly clerks and saleswomen). It was noted that the incidence of right shoulder pain and arm pain was significantly higher in cash register operators than in the other groups. Of interest was the high incidence too of symptoms such as fatigue, headache and insomnia, which suggested psychological stress. The incidence of OCD was reduced after the introduction of measures to limit keyboard operating hours and to introduce job rotation.

From Switzerland, Maeda *et al.* (1980) conducted a questionnaire comparison of the symptoms suggestive of OCD in female accounting machine operators with a control group of saleswomen in a department store, confining the study to subjects aged 17 to 29 years 'to remove from the obtained data the effects of such diseases as cervical spondylosis due to ageing' (*sic*). The researchers considered that there was a causal association between work activity and the increased prevalence of pain, stiffness and fatigue in the neck, arms and hands. There was a correlation between length of service and symptoms.

Luopajarvi *et al.* (1979) researched the prevalence of upper limb disorders in repetitive work in Finland. A significant increase in musculoskeletal disorders in the forearms and hands was found in assembly line packers compared with shop assistants.

Hocking (1987) contrasted the incidence of 'RSI' from data-based or accident reports and medical certificates in telephonists, clerical workers, telegraphists and process workers who worked for Telecom Australia. An 'epidemic' was described for the years 1981–85. The occupation most affected was that of telephonist (with a rate of 343 cases per 1000 keyboard staff over 5 years). The incidence in telegraphists was 34 per 1000 keyboard staff – in spite of their vastly greater keystroke rate per hour. No case of telegraphist's cramp was recorded. There was no increase with age and little evidence overall of a consistent dose–response relationship (leading the author to question the validity of a causal relationship between ergonomic factors and 'RSI').

Clinical features

Pain is the primary complaint. Although usually of insidious onset, it is acute or subacute in a significant number of patients, suggesting that a specific traumatic incident acted as the trigger. However, the description of relatively major trauma by patients is uncommon.

Initially symptoms are well localized, usually to the hand or wrist, although the neck or shoulder may be the primary site. In a subgroup of patients discomfort or 'numbness' radiates to one or more fingers. Pain or discomfort is relatively minor in severity, and resolves with rest, either overnight or at weekends. The symptoms are related to a particular task: in data processors this may involve the use of a keyboard mouse, whereas in process workers the manual task may be one small part of the operative process. There is no overt psychological disturbance of any severity at this stage.

Subsequently, the symptoms become more severe. The rate of progression is variable – sometimes a rapid worsening, but in other patients a gradual process over some months. It is not unusual for the initial symptoms to appear to resolve, only to recur at a later stage (for instance, within a few weeks or months), presumably stimulated by an additional stress. Pain becomes more constant and the sleep pattern is often disturbed. The symptoms are more extensive topographically – usually radiating proximally as far as the elbow, then the shoulder, neck and upper back (or, if commencing axially, radiating as 'referred' pain down the arm to the hand).

Pain often has a neuritic quality – described as burning, throbbing, stabbing, electric shock-like and aching. Sometimes it is cramping. Paraesthesiae are often felt in the fingers (in 91% in the series of Miller and Topliss, 1988). Frequently there is a subjective feeling of swelling, although this is not often observed clinically. Patients complain of weakness and occasionally of tenderness. One-quarter of Cohen's cases developed bilateral symptoms – though the symptoms in the non-dominant arm are usually less severe.

There is increasing intrusion into work, domestic and recreational activities. Loss of functional independence for a wide range of tasks becomes increasingly manifest. Psychological symptoms such as depression, headaches, disturbed sleep pattern and fatigue are frequently profound. Symptoms of distress and depression are reactive to pain and disability, often compounded by the transparent absence of medical curiosity about the condition that may suggest a personality disorder or neurosis to a busy practitioner. Features of abnormal illness behaviour may develop too but are not inevitable and, when present, should be viewed as a complication of neurosensitization, arising from a background of iatrogenic and sociocultural factors.

In the established case there is often a history of unsuccessful surgery for suspected carpal tunnel syndrome, for epicondylitis, or for de Quervain's tenovaginitis.

Examination findings

In the well-established case allodynia, hyperalgesia and hyperpathia are detected in multiple sites throughout the affected upper limb: these features are pathognomonic of neural sensitization. Mechanical hyperalgesia is evident as tender (or 'trigger') points in the muscles, and as articular discomfort on provocative stretching of the spinal and peripheral joints. There may be evidence of abnormal illness behaviour, such as the use of pain gestures to indicate suffering, and slow dysco-ordinated movements on attempting simple tasks (Selfe, 1995). The following features are frequently present.

Posture

An antalgic attitude of the upper limb gradually develops (Figure 6.1*a*). The elbow, wrist and fingers are held in flexion. There are few spontaneous movements of the hand or arm. As the condition usually affects the dominant arm, the patient may be disinclined to shake hands: at best, a very limp hand is proferred (Figure 6.1*b*).

Cervicodorsal spine

The signs of somatic dysfunction are commonly found in the cervical or proximal thoracic spines. These include segmental hypomobility, manifesting as loss of joint play (accessory movements) at the intervertebral joints, palpable hypertonus in the paravertebral muscles, spinous process tenderness and trigger points in the trapezii or proximal scapular fixator muscles.

Detection of many of these features requires experience in the examination of the spine for evidence of disturbed segmental function. Conventional orthopaedic examination, in which the only assessment of the cervicodorsal spine is an estimate of the range of active movements of the neck in the standing position, is inadequate. Should a relatively cursory examination of the cervical spine of this type be conducted, a minimal requirement is an assessment of end-feel (the sensation experienced by the examiner at the end of range): a feeling of stretching a piece of elastic at the end-range of some, not all, of the neck movements is commonly found.

Hypertonus of the suboccipital muscles, which is often associated with occipital headaches, may be present. Hypertonus of the paravertebral muscles overlying the apophyseal joints is most commonly detected at the C5–6 and C6–7 levels. In the thoracic spine, dysfunctional lesions at D3 and D4 are commonly found: spinous process tenderness is the most reliable sign. A marked feature in virtually all cases is hyperalgesia on firm palpation of the proximal scapular fixator muscles at the superomedial border of the scapula.

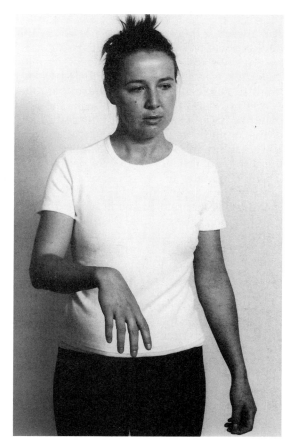

(a)

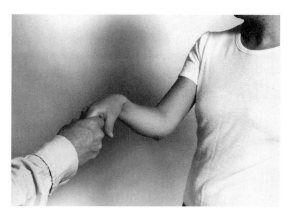

(b)

Figure 6.1 (*a*) A characteristic antalgic attitude of the upper limb is demonstrated in a patient with established neuropathic arm pain. (*b*) A very limp handshake is characteristic

Brachial plexus tension test (BPTT)

The brachial plexus tension test (BPTT), devised by Elvey (1986), is used particularly by physiotherapists with an interest in spinal disorders (see Figure 7.36). It helps to distinguish between shoulder and arm pain that is due to neural irritation and arm/shoulder pain that arises from lesions of the soft tissues of the shoulder region. It is a useful addition to the standard orthopaedic examination in the differential diagnosis of arm pain.

Unfortunately, in the presence of neural sensitization, as in type 2 WRULD, the interpretation of neural tension tests is difficult. Conduction of the brachial plexus tension test provokes mechanoreceptor activation in the musculotendinous and peri-articular soft tissues as well as neural tension throughout the limb. As a result, unless the patient is relaxed and has confidence in the skills of the doctor or therapist, the discriminant value of the test may be lost. In my view, although discomfort is usually experienced by the patient with type 2 WRULD on the conventional brachial plexus tension test, the presence of neural tension in the neck or arm should only be diagnosed if the requirement of patient relaxation is met.

Shoulder

The signs of subacromial dysfunction are frequently found. Active abduction of the affected arm at the shoulder is inhibited: both a painful arc and loss of terminal abduction are commonly present. Passive glenohumeral abduction and rotational movements are of full range although internal rotation is often uncomfortable terminally. The impingement sign is usually negative. Passive adduction is often uncomfortable and may be limited in range. There are no definite clinical abnormalities of the rotator cuff – a mild degree of diffuse weakness is common but there are no signs to indicate specific tendinopathy.

Palpable tenderness of the subacromial region is common. This does not usually extend to the acromioclavicular joint unless there is coincidental acromioclavicular joint pathology. Tenderness of the anterior chest wall medial to the shoulder (as described by Smythe, see Figure 5.34) may be detected.

Hyperalgesia

Diffuse hyperalgesia of muscles and joints is a feature of neuropathic arm pain (Figure 6.2). The muscle groups that are very frequently affected are: the cervical paravertebral muscles, the proximal scapular fixators, the pectorals, the common extensor and common flexor muscles of the proximal forearm, and the muscles in the first web space of the hand. The most characteristic (minimal) combination of muscle and joint tenderness is tenderness overlying the cervical apophyseal joints, in the superomedial scapular region, over the subacromial bursa anteriorly, in the common extensor muscles of the forearm approximately 6 cm distal to the lateral epicondyle, and over the radial aspect of the wrist.

The discomfort experienced by a patient for some time after a thorough musculoskeletal examination is a manifestation of hyperpathia.

Autonomic dysfunction

A subgroup of patients have a cold, swollen, blue hand, simulating the early stage of reflex sympathetic dystrophy (RSD). Sudomotor changes (manifesting usually as increased sweating) may also be evident. However, the more extensive (late stage) characteristics of RSD are not observed in type 2 WRULD, unless RSD subsequently arises as a complication of surgery (for suspected carpal tunnel syndrome, for instance) in those patients already sensitized.

Sensory phenomena

Patients commonly complain of sensory phenomena, including numbness and tingling. In my experience, however, evaluation of sensory loss is unrewarding. Should a comprehensive sensory examination be conducted, there is commonly loss of two point discrimination and variable but relatively minor loss of pin-prick/touch. This type of examination often provokes the onset of dysaesthesiae. Allodynia is extremely common, considered by some neurophysiologists to be an absolute criterion for the diagnosis of a neurogenic disorder.

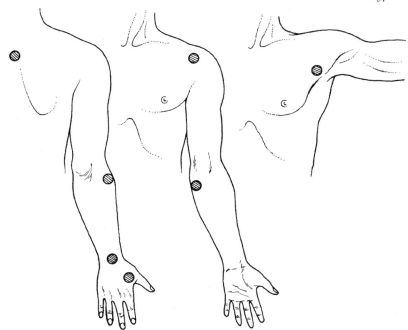

Figure 6.2 Widespread hyperalgesia is a feature of neuropathic arm pain. The characteristic sites are illustrated. A comparison may be made with Smythe's tender points in cervical syndromes (illustrated in Figure 5.34)

Dystonic and motor phenomena

Dystonic phenomena, such as poor coordination, cramps, fatigue on repetitive movements and loss of fine movements, occur in a subgroup of patients. Motor weakness is a ubiquitous finding in the hand and arm. However, there is no specific motor palsy and no significant muscle wasting.

Investigations

Should conventional investigations be conducted they are invariably negative. In particular, nerve conduction studies and electromyogram studies are normal. X-rays of the cervicordorsal spine reveal age-related changes only. Radionucleotide investigations reveal no increased uptake, and CT or MRI scanning techniques of the arm or cervicordorsal spine are negative.

Classification

Browne *et al.* (1984) classified 'RSI' on the basis of its increasing severity. They suggested

that stage 1 may be recognized by 'aching and tiredness', stage 2 by sleep disturbances and more persistent symptoms that become increasingly intrusive, and stage 3 by symptoms which persist at rest and last from months to years. Physical signs (which were not specified by Browne) were stated to be a variable feature of stage 2 but present consistently in stage 3. 'Increased muscle tension associated with mental stress' was noted to be a factor in the development of 'RSI'.

Although Browne's classification has been criticized, somewhat harshly in my view, for giving the impression that progression through the stages is inevitable if patients continue to subject themselves to provocative stresses, it was a useful contemporaneous contribution to the study of outcomes. It appeared dated as soon as the concept of RSI as a chronic pain syndrome emerged (Wright, 1987).

Pheasant (1994) has categorized WRULD into seven types. Type 1 includes the specific disorders described in Chapter 5 in this text. Pheasant's type 2 (which he calls the 'disseminated overuse syndrome') is the same as the regional pain syndrome – type 2 WRULD – described in this chapter. Pheasant's types 3 to 7 involve a combination of both type 1 and type 2. Whilst I agree with Pheasant that it is not uncommon for patients to develop disseminated symptoms as a consequence of a discrete type 1 condition, I do not feel that it is particularly helpful to subgroup these conditions as extensively as this.

My interpretation of the apparent metamorphosis from a discrete condition to a more diffuse condition in some cases is that either the initial type 1 diagnosis was incorrect, or that neural sensitization has occurred as a consequence. I favour the latter interpretation. This fits in particularly well with the hypothesis of Cohen *et al.* (1992) in which a soft tissue injury (as opposed to the more narrow concept of a neural injury) may be the trigger in some patients to the development of peripheral and central nervous system sensitization.

Hunter Fry has also categorized what he describes as 'overuse syndrome' of the upper limb in musicians into grades 1–5 (Dennett and Fry, 1988). Although I consider that Fry is mistaken in his choice of chronic muscle injury to explain the pathogenesis of conditions that are probably the same as those labelled type 2 WRULD in this text, it is noteworthy that his clinical observations include a significant loss of function in the limb and rest pain in grades 3, 4 and 5 (that suggest the development of a chronic pain syndrome).

Medical competence

A competent musculoskeletal examination is dependent upon two clinical criteria: (a) appropriate (manual medicine) expertise; (b) an interest and experience in functional disturbances of the musculoskeletal and neurological systems. If engaged in medicolegal work, clinicians may need to defend their views robustly when faced with the criticism that is sometimes levelled of lack of objectivity (*sic*), particularly with respect to the identification and interpretation of allodynia and hyperalgesia. Physical signs demand an explanation: the oft-heard rejection of an organic basis (in favour of neurosis or malingering) for type 2 WRULD on the basis of 'inappropriate' signs assumes at worst an arrogance associated

with medical authoritarianism or at best a Nelsonian (blind eye) attitude towards the experimental work and literature on chronic pain mechanisms and their practical manifestations that have emerged over the recent decade or two.

The credibility of the 'structuralist' demand for histopathological evidence of 'disease' in type 2 WRULD will diminish as the recognition of the neural pathogenesis of chronic pain syndromes becomes more established. In a state of the art review entitled 'Psychological and physical aspects of occupational arm pain' (1988), Ireland's brief description of the examination findings in a typical case comprised the following:

This [upper limb] pain, although often consistent in a given patient, is not consistent between patients and does not conform to any known neurological pathway, anatomical structure or physiological pattern. There are no primary objective physical findings in the upper limbs other than tenderness which is frequently of equal severity at any randomly selected point on the limb. . . . There are no sequelae of tissue trauma such as swelling, bruising, redness or increased temperature.

The prescience of Sir Francis Walshe may yet be redeemed: rescue is surely to hand.

Management principles

Type 2 WRULD: early

At this stage the condition is potentially reversible. Appropriate therapeutic measures are based on counselling, reduction of stressors and the modification of the afferent barrage to the central nervous system. An essential aspect is individualized treatment, which is summarized as follows.

- **Containment (prevention of progression)**
  early diagnosis
  appropriate explanation to patient
  avoidance of iatrogenesis (requires musculoskeletal medical expertise)
  identification of work risk factors
- **Modification of work risk factors**
  ergonomic assessment

job rotation
cessation of overtime
reduction of work rate
increase in rest periods
liaison with senior work personnel
technical assessment (musicians particularly)

- **Symptomatic relief**
  acupuncture
  acupressure
  TENS
  trigger point therapy
  – massage
  – injection
  – stretching (Figure 6.3)
  – rest, if indicated
- **Physical treatment of underlying dysfunction**
  nerve root mobilization (nerve decompression)
  spinal joint mobilization (relief of somatic dysfunction)
  neural blockade
  – 'sinuvertebral' blocks
  – facet blocks (Figure 6.4)
  trigger point therapy
- **Relaxation**
  frequent brief relaxation at work (Wigley, 1990)
  massage
  physical conditioning exercise programme
- **Psychological**
  stress counselling
  restoration of sleep pattern
  restoration of positive attitudes
  tricyclics

Type 2 WRULD: established

It is generally accepted that therapies predicated on conventional disease entities, and strategies predicated on conventional disease–illness models, are uniformly unsuccessful. Treatments directed solely at reducing nociceptor activation at the site of tissue injury are inadequate, as the pain mechanisms are driven by low threshold mechanoreceptor afferents.

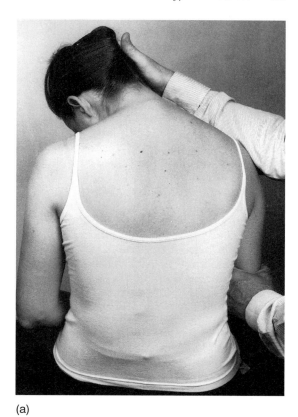

(a)

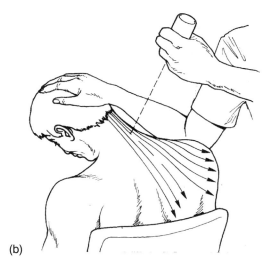

(b)

Figure 6.3 Effective management of a trigger point should include a stretching regimen. (*a*) Stretching of the proximal scapular fixator muscles is demonstrated by the examiner. (*b*) A vapocoolant spray may be used to inhibit the trigger point. (After Travell and Simons, 1983)

Neuropathic arm pain (NAP)
- Education of patient (and employer)
- Ergonomic improvements
- Relaxation therapies
- Symptomatic relief
- Tricyclics
- Rehabilitation counselling

Neuropathic arm pain (NAP) and abnormal illness behaviour (AIB)
- Cognitive-behavioural therapy

Spinal injection techniques

When the source of neck and arm pain is considered to be at the spinal level (or when it is considered likely that a significant contribution to arm pain is from spinal disturbance), injection blockade in experienced hands is a useful adjunct to therapy.

Test blockades with local anaesthetic may be performed for diagnostic and prognostic purposes (Stolker, 1994); ideally, therapeutic blockade should then be based upon the result of a previous diagnostic blockade. In practice, an empiric management strategy may include the use of a combined steroid and local anaesthetic blockade at one or more spinal levels following a sound clinical examination.

The choice of blockade is dependent upon the target structure. Logically, a facet syndrome may be treated by a **medial branch** (of the dorsal ramus) **block** or by an (intra-articular) **facet block**; in the cervical spine a nerve block is probably the safest (Figure 6.4). The clinical criteria include: paravertebral and/or referred pain, segmental hypomobility, paravertebral muscle tenderness and hypertonus, positive articular signs (for instance, pain on ipsilateral rotation).

If nerve root compression or irritation is diagnosed, a periradicular or sinuvertebral block is desirable. However, periradicular blocks in the cervical spine suffer from the practical disadvantage of requiring fluoroscopic screening, and selective sinuvertebral blocks are virtually impossible (without overflow to the sympathetic chain and spinal nerves). In my experience (anecdotal, without a control group), a pragmatic strategy in the cervical spine is the infiltration of the posterior aspects of adjacent facet joints with low-dose steroid and local anaesthetic – a technique that may yield good results in both

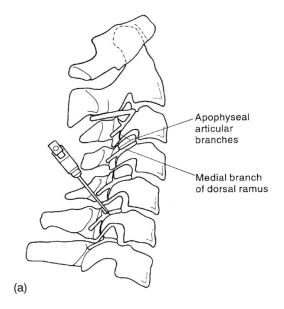

Apophyseal articular branches

Medial branch of dorsal ramus

(a)

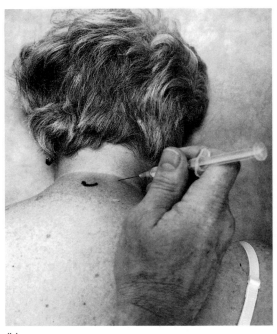

(b)

Figure 6.4 Neural blockade, in the form of medial branch block injections, is often helpful in chronic facet joint dysfunction. (*a*) Diagrammatic representation of a C6 medial branch block. (After Lord *et al.*, 1993). (*b*) The technique is demonstrated with the patient prone: the angle of needle penetration is slightly lateral to medial. The skin marker denotes the position of C7 spinous process

dorsal (facet joint) syndromes and ventral (root entrapment) syndromes.

Clearly, individual assessment of patients with established neuropathic arm pain is necessary prior to contemplation of neural blockade. This management strategy may be utilized in those patients (the majority) in whom there are clinical features that suggest a nociceptive source or a pain-maintaining locus in the cervical spine. Pain relief following a medial branch block may also indicate a placebo response or an (overflow) myogenic block. Whatever the mechanism, partial pain relief may be experienced for longer than the duration of the local anaesthetic if several treatments are given over a 6–8 week period. **For patients with neuropathic arm pain, I have found that the most effective physical therapy is the combination of neural blocks and neural mobilization.**

Tricyclic antidepressants

Tricyclic antidepressants are the drugs of choice for neuropathic pain. Amitriptyline is probably the most widely used, but other drugs such as doxepin and dothiepin are available. The mechanism of action is thought to be mediated through 5-hydroxytryptamine (5-HT) and noradrenaline descending systems originating in the brain stem and acting upon the dorsal horn of the spinal cord (Charlton, 1993).

The starting dose is 10 mg amitriptyline at night, increasing by small increments every two weeks. The dosage may need to be increased to 50–100 mg. A helpful side effect is the improved sleep pattern, but a dry mouth and diurnal drowsiness are frequently troublesome.

Treatment should not be abandoned because of apparent lack of early response; patients should be advised that it may take some time to establish reasonable pain relief. Therapy should then continue for some considerable time, dependent upon the overall progress and subject to regular monitoring.

Alternative analgesic regimes include the development of neurokinin and NMDA receptor inhibitors which may prove to be safer for routine use than the powerful endogenous opioids (Kidd *et al.*, 1996).

Cognitive-behavioural therapy

Patients with chronic pain may learn maladaptive behavioural patterns; if illness behaviour becomes a dominant feature, modification of these patterns through learning is often an effective treatment. Patients are disabused of the concepts that 'pain means injury' and 'if it hurts, stop', as these contribute to chronicity. Treatment strategies are directed towards increased functional activity, increased functional independence, and the transfer of the control of pain and its associated problems to the patient. An important goal is reduction of the self-report of pain intensity. (Patients often consider pain to be the most important reference point with respect to the severity of their condition and progress.) Unfortunately, the benefits from improvements in activity levels and other outcome measures may be reversed by over-sympathetic responses from spouses, friends, family members and physicians to the complaint of persistent pain (Keefe *et al.*, 1981).

Cognitive-behavioural therapy was pioneered by Fordyce and his colleagues in the USA (Fordyce, 1973). Keefe emphasized the importance of relaxation procedures when treating a series of patients with low back pain in Durham, NC (USA). Williams *et al.* (1993) treated 212 patients with chronic pain at St Thomas' Hospital, London, by an inpatient programme ('INPUT') which involved a multidisciplinary team. The principal components of their cognitive-behavioural therapy included: education, teaching behavioural and cognitive skills, a stretch and exercise programme, medication reduction, goal setting and pacing, and relaxation training. Significant improvements in all outcome measures were recorded; improvements were well maintained at 6-month follow-up.

Joyce Williams (1989) has reported on the success of the 'School for Bravery' approach to patients with chronic pain – a combination of behaviour modification and exercise in an active physiotherapy gymnasium. The excellent results overall (converting 'illness behaviour' to 'wellness behaviour') were adversely affected by those patients who experienced financial gain or were seeking compensation as a result of injury.

References

Armstrong, T.J. and Chaffin, D. (1979) Carpal tunnel syndrome and selected personal attributes. *J. Occup. Med.*, **21**, 481–6.

Arroyo, J.F. and Cohen, M.L. (1992) Unusual responses to electrocutaneous stimulation in refractory cervicobrachial pain: clues to a neuropathic pathogenesis. *Clin. Exp. Rheumatol.*, **10**, 475–82.

Browne, C.D., Nolan, B.M. and Faithfull, D.K. (1984) Occupational repetition strain injuries: guidelines to diagnosis and management. *Med. J. Aust.*, **140**, 329–32.

Charlton, E. (1993) Neuropathic pain, *Prescribers' J.*, **33**(6), 244–9.

Cohen, M.L., Arroyo, J.F., Champion, G.D. and Browne, C.D. (1992) In search of the pathogenesis of refractory cervicobrachial pain syndrome. *Med. J. Aust.*, **156**, 432–6.

Dennett, X. and Fry, H.J.H. (1988) Overuse syndrome: a muscle biopsy study. *Lancet*, **i**, 905–8.

Elvey, R.L. (1986) Treatment of arm pain associated with abnormal brachial plexus tension. *Aust. J. Physiother.*, **32**, 225–30.

Fordyce, W.E. (1973). *Behavioural Methods for Chronic Pain and Illness.* C.V. Mosby, St Louis, MO.

Helme, R.D., Gibson, S.J. and Khalil, Z. (1990) Neural pathways in chronic pain. *Med. J. Aust.*, **153**, 400–406.

Hocking, B. (1987). Epidemiological aspects of 'repetition strain injury' in Telecom Australia. *Med. J. Aust.*, **147**, 218–22.

Ireland, D.C.R. (1988) Psychological and physical aspects of occupational arm pain. *J. Hand Surg.*, **13B**(1), 5–10.

Karlsson, J. and Ollander, B. (1972) Muscle metabolites with exhaustive static exercise of different durations. *Acta Physiol. Scand.*, **86**, 309–14.

Keefe, F.J., Block, A.R., Williams, R.B. and Surwit, R.S. (1981). Behavioural treatment of chronic low back pain: clinical outcome and individual differences in pain relief. *Pain*, **11**, 221–31.

Kidd, B.L., Morris, V.H. and Urban, L. (1966) Pathophysiology of joint pain. *Ann. Rheum. Dis.*, **55**, 276–83.

Lord, S., Barnsley, L. and Bogduk, N. (1993) Cervical zygapophyseal joint pain in whiplash. *Spine, State Art Rev.*, **7**(3), 355–72.

Luopajarvi, T., Kuorinka, I., Virolainen, M. and Holmberg, M. (1979) Prevalence of tenosynovitis and other injuries of the upper extremities in repetitive work. *Scand. J. Work Environ. Health*, **5**(3), 48–55.

McDermott, F.T. (1986) Repetition strain injury: a review of current understanding. *Med. J. Aust.*, **144**, 196–200.

Maeda, K., Hunting, W. and Grandjean, E. (1980) Localised fatigue in accounting-machine operators, *J. Occup. Med.*, **22**(12), 810–16.

Miller, M.H. and Topliss, D.J. (1988) Chronic upper limb pain syndrome (repetitive strain injury) in the Australian workforce: a systematic cross sectional rheumatological study of 229 patients. *J. Rheumatol.*, **15**(11), 1705–12.

Pell, R. (1994) Painful regional occupational disorder. *J. Orthop. Med.*, **16**(2), 57–63.

Pheasant, S.T. (1992) Does RSI exist? *J. Occup. Med.*, **42**, 167–8.

Pheasant, S.T. (1994) Repetitive strain injury – towards a clarification of the points at issue. *J. Personal Injury Litigation*, September, pp. 223–30.

Raffle, P.A.B. *et al.* (1994) Repetitive strain syndrome. In: *Hunter's Diseases of Occupations*, 8th edn., pp. 520–27. E. Arnold, London.

Rathbun, J.B. and McNab, I. (1970) The microvascular pattern of the rotator cuff. *J. Bone Joint. Surg.*, **52B**, 540–53.

Selfe, J. (1995) Abnormal illness behaviours in chronic back pain: a practical guide. *J. Orthop. Med.*, **17**(1), 27–8.

Sharma, S.D., Smith, E.M., Hazleman, B.L. and Jenner, J.R. (1977) Thermographic changes in keyboard operators with chronic forearm pain. *Br. Med. J.*, **314**, 118.

Stolker, R.J., Vervest, A.C.M. and Groen, G.J. (1994) The management of chronic spinal pain by blockades: a review. *Pain*, **58**, 1–20.

Travell, J.G. and Simons, D.G. (1983) *The Trigger Point Manual.* Williams & Wilkins, Baltimore, MD.

Walshe, F.M.R. (1945) On 'acroparaesthesia' and so-called 'neuritis' of the hands and arms in women. *Br. Med. J.*, **2**, 596–8.

Wigley, R.D. (1990) Repetitive strain syndrome – fact not fiction. *NZ Med. J.*, **103**, 75–6.

Williams, A.C. de C, Nicholas, M.K., Richardson, P.H. and Pither, C.E. (1993) Evaluation of a cognitive behavioural programme for rehabilitating patients with chronic pain. *Br. J. Gen. Pract.*, **43**, 513–18.

Williams, J.I. (1989) Illness behaviour to wellness behaviour: the 'School for Bravery' approach. *Physiotherapy*, **75**(1), 2–7.

Wright, G.D. (1987) The failure of the 'RSI' concept. *Med. J. Aust.*, **147**, 233–6.

7

Musculoskeletal examination

Moreover, if the diagnosis is made early, before the inevitable delays in reaching an appropriate pain clinic, perhaps some patients may be saved from the stigma of being mistakenly labelled as 'neurotic' or 'hysterical', and the secondary psychological and socio-economic effects caused by suffering chronic pain of unknown origin might be averted.

Bogduk and Marsland (1988)

The neck and upper back, shoulder girdles, shoulders, arms and hands are examined. Musculoskeletal examination of the upper limb (as elsewhere in the body) is predicated on the recognition that disorders may be degenerative, inflammatory, neoplastic, infective or dysfunctional. Assessment of function is a particularly important aspect of the examination.

The nervous system should also be examined carefully for functional disturbances which may affect one or more of its components – central, peripheral and autonomic. Topographically, function of one part of the limb, for instance the hand, can only be fully evaluated if the rest of the limb, the axial skeleton and the contralateral limb are examined.

General features

The patient's demeanour when accepting the examiner's friendly handshake at the beginning of the interview is a relevant clinical sign. Patients may have become accustomed to protecting their hand/upper limb as a result of their painful disorder, and a weak, limp handshake is typical of type 2 WRULD in particular (see Figure 6.1b). Indeed, a firm, positive handshake, hardly ever found when assessing patients with WRULD of any type, is a strong pointer against its diagnosis.

Whilst wishing to allow the patient a modicum of decorum and privacy during undressing for the examination, much information may be gained from its observation. A note may be made of the manner in which the arms are used, and of difficulties experienced during intricate manoeuvres, such as manipulating buttons. Pain gestures and the slow, somewhat dysco-ordinated movements that are typical of abnormal illness behaviour may also be observed. For similar reasons, discomfort and difficulty on dressing at the conclusion of the examination should be noted: by this stage patients with abnormal illness behaviour may feel 'exhausted', and patients with neuropathic pain may complain of increased discomfort.

During a general examination the systemic manifestations of diseases such as rheumatoid arthritis and myxoedema are recorded. Allodynia and hyperalgesia are noted. Widespread muscle tenderness and discomfort on stretching the joint capsules and periarticular connective tissues are likely to be expressions of mechanical hyperalgesia. Although there is no universal agreement on terminology for tender, hypertonic muscles, it is generally accepted that such semi-objective clinical signs are valid findings. It should be noted that 'trigger points', 'tender points' and 'hyperalgesic muscle' are all in common usage.

According to Travell, a *trigger* point combines extreme tenderness (manifesting as the 'jump sign') and a palpable taut band (Travell and Simons, 1983). Effectively, the muscle is shortened. Trigger points in the trapezii and the proximal scapular fixator muscles are commonly found in structural and functional disturbances of the cervical spine. Trigger points in the arm should also be noted, and an attempt made subsequently to correlate these findings with other clinical signs, such as adverse neural tension.

Muscles that do not exhibit the jump sign may be tender and apparently hypertonic. These *tender points* should also be recorded. Tenderness and hypertonicity in the strap muscles of the cervical spine and in the muscles of the arms should be considered to be areas of secondary hyperalgesia when widespread. They are a cardinal feature of type 2 WRULD, occurring frequently in the cervical paravertebral musculature, in the proximal scapular fixators, in the common extensor and flexor muscles of the forearm, and in the web between the thumb and the forefinger.

The cervical spine

A comprehensive clinical examination for the detection of the plethora of conditions that comprise the work-related upper limb disorders must include the cervical spine. Indeed, it is a logical place to start. When pain is felt in the neck or shawl area the differential diagnosis includes cervical intervertebral disc disease, somatic (reversible) spinal joint dysfunction, primary muscle hypertonus and secondary hyperalgesia. Discomfort in the neck may be a relatively minor symptom, but its significance is likely to be profound.

Observation
Occasionally, patients are seen with a torticollis, which in adults may be due to a cervical intervertebral disc prolapse, but which also may be 'hysterical'. However, in the context of the conditions being considered in this text, it is more usual for the posture of the head and neck to be substantially normal, without obvious spasm of the sternomastoid. The cervical lordosis may be accentuated and the head protracted as a result of a thoracic kyphosis (arising, for instance, from poor posture,

Scheuermann's disease, or degenerative changes in the thoracic spine).

Active and passive movements
Observation of the alignment of the cervical spine is followed by a study of the *active* movements of the neck in the standing or sitting position. Forward flexion, extension, side flexions to right and left, and rotations to right and left are the movements examined. The range of movement and pain, if present, are noted. Gentle overpressure by the examiner at the end of range provides an assessment of the *passive* movements and the end-feel.

The reaction of the patient to *gentle* overpressure is also an indicator of the patient's 'state of mind': a dramatic reaction associated with a very protective attitude may indicate abnormal illness behaviour, although articular mechanoreceptor stimulation may also evoke increased discomfort in patients with chronic pain (an example of mechanical hyperalgesia). A 'twingey' end-feel is found with an articular disturbance.

When recording the cervical movements, a diagram of the type illustrated in Figure 7.1 may be useful: it allows for an estimate of pain as well as the range of movement. Care should be exercised when identifying 'loss' of mobility, as the normal range varies from individual to individual. A valid criticism of an examiner's record of 'half normal range' is that the premorbid range is commonly assumed but probably unknown.

Cervical rotation is usually considered to be within the range 70–90 degrees, but by the sixth decade of life painless rotation (with bone-on-bone end-feel) is often reduced to 45–60 degrees. Flexion usually approximates to 90 degrees, the chin abutting the chest at full range; flexion is often well maintained in cervical spondylosis (unlike the other movements) so painful loss of flexion is significant. Extension usually has an empty end-feel as there is no anatomical block to movement – hence the profound articular disturbance found after whiplash in which there is uncontrolled hyperextension. Pain on extension may indicate a lesion at the cervicodorsal junction (when the other movements are relatively pain-free) or a lesion situated more proximally in the mid-cervical spine (when some of the other movements are painful).

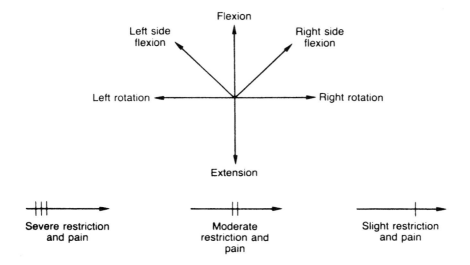

Figure 7.1 A diagrammatic representation of the movements of the cervical spine facilitates the recording of pain and/or loss of passive range of movement. (From Hutson, 1993)

Side flexions are usually 25–40 degrees in range. It is not unusual to find that side flexion away from the painful side is uncomfortable if there is tension within the trapezius muscle. On the other hand, painful ipsilateral side flexion or rotation suggests an articular disturbance at the apophyseal joint(s). The provocative test of combined passive extension and ipsilateral rotation is highly sensitive for the detection of nerve root irritation/compression at the intervertebral foramen: an increase in limb pain on this manoeuvre indicates neural compression (Figure 7.2).

Resisted (isometric) movements

Resisted contraction of the six movements already described may be performed with the neck in the neutral position. So long as no movement of the neck is allowed during the procedure, it is unusual for pain or weakness of isolated muscle groups to be identified.

Whilst the patient remains standing (or sitting), the function of the trapezii may be assessed by requesting the patient to shrug their shoulders against resistance. It is unusual to find either unilateral or bilateral weakness (which would indicate more serious pathology) and discomfort is infrequent. Active scapular movements and rotational movements of the trunk may also be assessed

at this stage (see below) prior to examination of the cervical spine with the patient in the supine position.

Joint play movements

With the patient supine, and the head held gently by the examiner's hands cupping the occiput, an assessment should be made of the accessory (joint play) movements (Figure 7.3). I recommend anteroposterior translation, side glidings to right and left, and side flexions to right and left. Additionally, the atlanto-occipital (C0–1) segment may be assessed by applying gentle side flexion when the neck is fully rotated.

Localized hypomobility on joint play assessment, often accompanied by discomfort, should be recorded: it indicates segmental dysfunction. The detection of hypomobility of the articulations between the atlas and the occiput, and the atlas and the axis, and dysfunctions of the upper ribs requires considerable experience in osteopathic manual techniques.

Palpation

Next, a note is made of spinous process tenderness. If present, this is more usually felt in the mid- and distal cervical spines. Muscle hypertonus should be palpated by the examiner's index, long and ring fingers whilst the

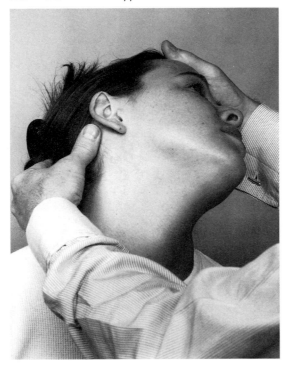

Figure 7.2 Combined extension and ipsilateral rotation of the cervical spine aggravates the radicular symptoms in nerve root compression

patient's cervical spine is fully relaxed in the supine position. Tension in the small suboccipital muscles is usually accompanied by a tactile sensation of swelling of the overlying soft tissues – probably due to subcutaneous oedema. Unilateral hypertonus is palpable in the strap muscles overlying the apophyseal joints in the presence of spinal joint dysfunction.

In a relaxed patient in the supine position, the anterolateral margins of the lower cervical intervertebral discs may be palpated for tenderness by gently introducing the thumb or the pulp pads of the examining fingers medial to the sternomastoid at the C5–6 level, and between the sternal and clavicular insertions of the sternomastoid at the C6–7 level (Figure 7.4).

Neurological assessment of the upper limbs is an important part of a comprehensive cervical spinal examination, and this is conducted at some stage when the patient returns to a standing or sitting position. The brachial

plexus tension test (BPTT) is best conducted whilst the patient is supine, but for convenience it is described below (see Neurological examination).

The shoulder girdles

The shoulder of the dominant arm generally appears lower than the non-dominant side. Muscle hypertrophy around the scapula and shoulder of the dominant arm may be obvious on inspection, and the scapula is often positioned further laterally from the spine.

In the standing position, the patient is asked actively to retract and protract their shoulder girdles. This demands active contraction of those muscles attached to the scapulae. Active retraction (by contraction of the trapezius, rhomboids and levator scapulae) may provoke discomfort felt in the medial scapular region (Figure 7.5). Protraction, which may be reinforced by overpressure from the examiner, gives rise to discomfort in the same region as a result of stretching of the same muscle groups. Gross weakness of the muscles attached to the scapula is unusual other than for winging of the scapula (weakness of serratus anterior due to a palsy of the long thoracic nerve of Bell). The phenomenon of pseudo-winging of the scapula during elevation of the arm is occasionally seen in a shoulder that is very unstable.

Further assessment of the tone of the muscles attached to the scapulae should be performed with the patient sitting. Increased tone in the proximal scapular fixator muscles is often associated with the appearance of asymmetry of the superomedial borders of the scapulae, possibly as a result of muscle spasm. Palpation of the scapular attachments of the proximal scapular fixator muscles (the trapezii and levator scapulae in particular) commonly reveals tenderness, hypertonus and a positive jump sign (indicating a 'trigger" point). This is a common finding in keyboard workers, when it is thought to reflect the static loading of these muscles. It may also occur in workers undertaking jobs that require frequent and repetitive use of the arms away from the sides of the body.

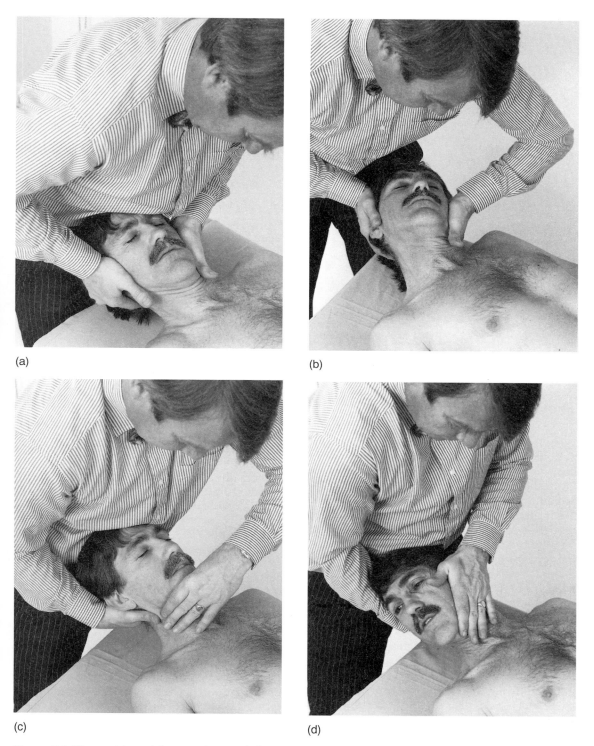

(a)

(b)

(c)

(d)

Figure 7.3 The position of the examiner and the patient are demonstrated for the assessment of joint play movements: (*a*) side gliding; (*b*) side bending; (*c*) anteroposterior translation; (*d*) atlanto-occipital rock

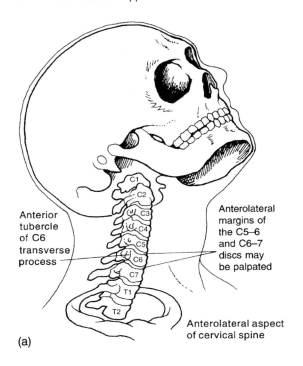

(a)

Anterior tubercle of C6 transverse process

Anterolateral margins of the C5–6 and C6–7 discs may be palpated

Anterolateral aspect of cervical spine

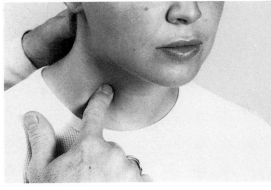

(b)

Figure 7.4 The anterolateral margins of the lower cervical intervertebral discs may be palpated by introducing the examining finger in front of or behind the sternomastoid muscle: (*a*) illustrated diagrammatically; (*b*) demonstrated clinically

Thoracic spine

When standing, or preferably sitting, the patient is asked to put their hands behind the back of their neck, interlocking their fingers, with the arms abducted. Alternatively, the patient may cross their arms diagonally across the front of their chest, placing their palms on the front of their shoulders. In this position, passive rotation of the trunk to the right and the left is undertaken (Figure 7.6). Although maximal rotational movement of the trunk takes place in the distal thoracic spine, nevertheless rotation to one side or the other often provokes discomfort if there is proximal or mid-thoracic spinal joint dysfunction. Occasionally, movement is restricted unilaterally.

When pain is felt in the back, for instance in the interscapular region, on passive neck flexion, significant segmental dysfunction of the spine, such as a disc prolapse causing dural irritation, should be suspected.

The patient is examined in the prone position, without a pillow and preferably with the neck in neutral (with the aid of a breathing slot in the couch). The signs of localized segmental dysfunction are sought (Hutson, 1993).

1 *Skin rolling*. The examiner should be familiar with the technique of palpation of altered skin texture. Positive skin rolling is detected by the presence of thickening of the skin and subcutaneous tissues, unilaterally or bilaterally, overlying the paravertebral muscles (Figure 7.7). Cutaneous tenderness, an expression of allodynia, may be experienced by the patient on gentle stroking of the skin. There may be underlying muscle hypertonus which, although stated by osteopathic physicians to be easy to detect, may be a relatively subtle sign in the thoracic region.

2 *Vertebral springing* is undertaken segmentally. The ulnar border of the hand (effectively, the fifth metacarpal) is used to produce localized hyperextension at each vertebral level. To control the movement, the examiner reinforces compression with the other hand (Figure 7.8*a*). Discomfort is recorded and an evaluation made of the degree of anteroposterior mobility. Segmental or regional hypomobility needs an explanation: for instance,

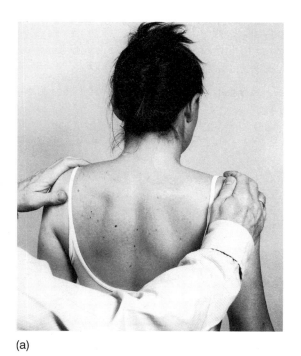

(a)

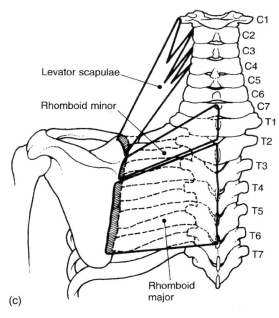

(c)

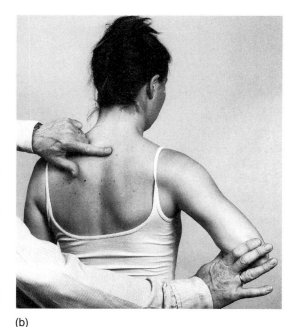

(b)

Figure 7.5 (*a*) Active retraction of the scapulae may provoke discomfort in the medial scapular region. (*b*) Rhomboid minor is demonstrated when the patient braces her right shoulder backwards against resistance. (*c*) Diagrammatic representation of the scapular fixators

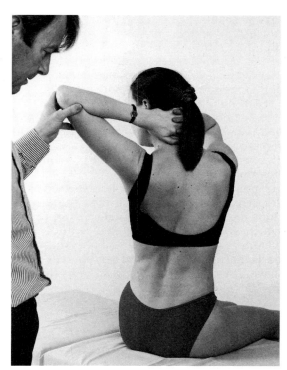

Figure 7.6 Passive rotation of the trunk is undertaken as a provocative test for thoracic spinal dysfunction

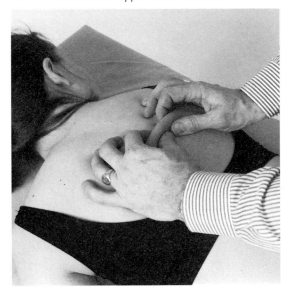

Figure 7.7 The technique of skin rolling is demonstrated. (From Hutson, 1993)

it could be due to degenerative changes over several segments, or to localized somatic dysfunction. Lateral pressure applied by the examiner's thumbs to the spinous processes of the upper thoracic spine is an additional method of evaluating segmental discomfort and tenderness (Figure 7.8*b*).

With the patient in the prone position, the opportunity is taken to perform skin rolling and vertebral springing throughout the dorsilumbar spine. Extensive allodynia and hyperalgesia may be found, raising the possibility of fibromyalgia. The presence of a unilateral trigger point in the glutei and tenderness of the adjacent posterior superior iliac spine indicates the possibility of sacroiliac dysfunction which is commonly associated with cervical or upper thoracic spinal joint dysfunction, particularly in keyboard operatives and machinists (and following rear-end vehicular collisions).

Shoulders

Observation

The shoulders should be inspected for deformities such as the step deformity associated with acromioclavicular joint (ACJ) dislocation. A previous injury such as this may

predispose to discomfort around the shoulder on repetitive forceful overhead work. Muscle wasting around the shoulder girdle may be localized – to the spinati, for instance, as a result of a rotator cuff tear – or more generalized, when it is often bilateral (indicating the

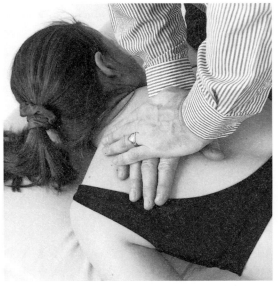

(a)

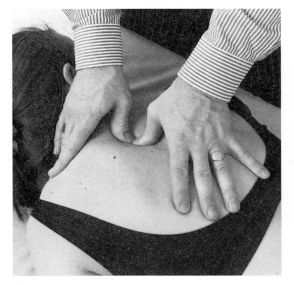

(b)

Figure 7.8 Segmental discomfort may be elicited by (*a*) vertebral springing and (*b*) lateral pressure upon the spinous process. (From Hutson, 1993)

possibility of neuralgic amyotrophy). Muscle wasting is not a feature of type 2 WRULD.

Active movements

Examination of the shoulder should continue by assessment of active abduction. This yields information about the function of the shoulder joint, the acromioclavicular joint, the sternoclavicular joint, the scapulothoracic 'joint', the subacromial 'joint' and the periarticular structures such as the rotator cuff. Additionally, it is not uncommon for patients with type 2 WRULD to experience discomfort in the arm as far as the hand on full active abduction of the arm (as an expression of mechanical hyperalgesia). Full abduction of both shoulders simultaneously may be uncomfortable and/or restricted if there is significant segmental dysfunction in the upper thoracic spine or as a consequence of a thoracic kyphosis (Figure 7.9).

An arc of pain on active abduction indicates subacromial impingement (Figure 7.10). Significant terminal loss of active abduction raises the possibility of capsulitis or other glenohumeral pathology. (A greater loss of external rotation than abduction or internal rotation will confirm the capsular pattern.) Pain during the terminal 10–15 degrees of abduction (but with a normal range of external rotation) suggests acromioclavicular joint dysfunction (Figure 7.11); if the acromioclavicular joint disorder is substantial, there is painful loss of the terminal 10 degrees of abduction too (Hutson, 1996).

Passive movements

The passive movements are best examined with the patient standing. The range of glenohumeral abduction is assessed by passively abducting the arm by the elbow whilst holding the inferior border of the scapula down with the other hand. External rotation should be assessed when the examiner stands close to the patient, fixing the elbow and rotating the forearm (Figure 7.12). Internal rotation should be assessed by identifying how far the dorsum of the patient's hand or forefinger may be brought up their back (Figure 7.13).

Passive horizontal adduction is performed by gently adducting the arm across the chest: this is a particularly useful and sensitive test for acromioclavicular joint function (Figure

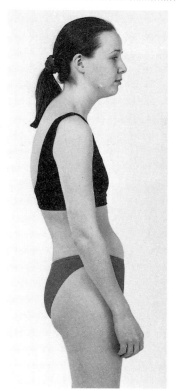

Figure 7.9 Poor spinal posture gives rise to round shoulders, thoracic kyphosis and compensatory cervical hyperextension. Active abduction of the shoulders is often impaired. (From Hutson, 1993)

7.14). Painful loss of full adduction indicates acromioclavicular joint pathology.

The impingement test is performed by the combination of forward flexion of the arm to 90 degrees and internal rotation with the elbow bent to 90 degrees (Figure 7.15). This is painful in subacromial impingement but far less commonly so in subacromial dysfunction that is secondary to spinal dysfunction. Terminal discomfort on forward flexion of the arm at the shoulder is also a sign of subacromial impingement.

Resisted (isometric) movements

The rotator cuff is assessed by resisted (isometric) contraction. Resisted abduction, resisted external rotation and resisted internal rotation of the shoulder are undertaken. When examined sequentially and followed by resisted flexion of the elbow, these assess the function of the supraspinatus, infraspinatus,

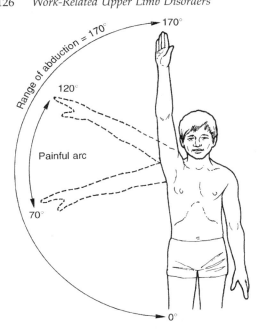

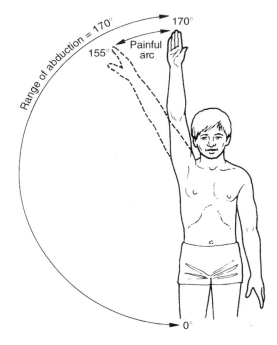

Figure 7.10 The painful arc of subacromial impingement

Figure 7.11 Acromioclavicular painful arc: pain during the terminal 10–15 degrees of abduction (with a normal range of external rotation) suggests acromioclavicular joint dysfunction

subscapularis and biceps brachii respectively (Figure 7.16). The examiner notes the presence of pain and weakness.

It is common to find painful weakness of resisted abduction, indicating a chronic supraspinatus tendinitis, in patients who subject their rotator cuffs to overload when the arms are held repetitively or for prolonged periods in abduction, flexion and internal rotation. (Poor work postures may be the cause.) This is often associated with tenderness at the insertion of the supraspinatus tendon on to the greater tuberosity of the humerus.

Joint play and tests for instability
Occasionally, in manual workers who are accustomed to exerting considerable force at or above shoulder level, for instance those workers engaged in stacking car tyres by throwing them into overhead racks (Figure 7.17), glenohumeral instability may be symptomatic. The type of instability that is manifest under these circumstances is often a chronic, recurrent, involuntary, multidirectional subluxation that may be very disabling and difficult to treat.

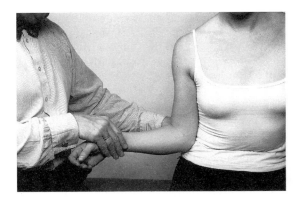

Figure 7.12 Passive external rotation at the shoulder is demonstrated: the patient's elbow is held close to the side of her body

With respect to aetiology, it is sometimes difficult to differentiate between cause and effect, particularly when patients have been accustomed over several years to other activities that are also stressful for the shoulder,

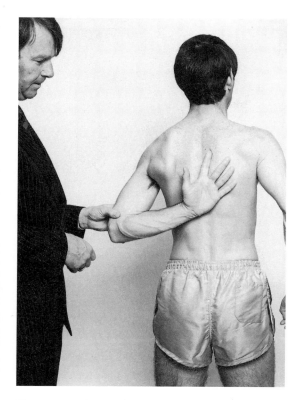

Figure 7.13 Internal rotation may be assessed by identifying the level at which the dorsum of the patient's hand or forefinger reaches up the back

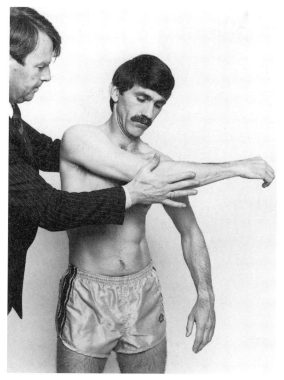

Figure 7.14 Passive horizontal adduction is a particularly useful provocative test for the acromioclavicular joint

such as cricket or tennis in addition to repeated overhead work. If glenohumeral instability is suspected, the appropriate tests for anterior, posterior and inferior instability are performed. The presence of glenohumeral laxity in the non-involved shoulder or in several other joints as well as the painful shoulder raises the possibility of the hypermobility syndrome. At the very least, multi-joint laxity indicates a constitutional predisposition to painful joint strains or symptomatic instability.

Inferior laxity may be demonstrated by the sulcus sign when the examiner exerts downward traction on the arm (Figure 7.18*a*). The anterior apprehension test for anterior instability may be performed with the patient standing, sitting or lying. When in the supine position, this test may be augmented by the demonstration of abnormal anterior translation of the head of the humerus (Figure 7.18*b*). The Jobe relocation test is then usually positive: backwards pressure on the neck of the

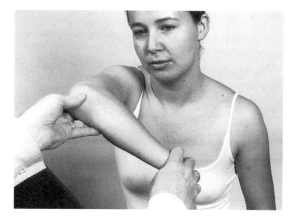

Figure 7.15 The impingement test (for subacromial impingement) is performed by the combination of forward flexion of the arm to 90 degrees and internal rotation with the elbow flexed to 90 degrees

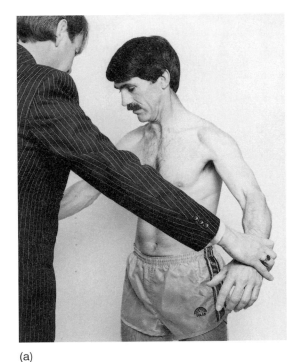

(a)

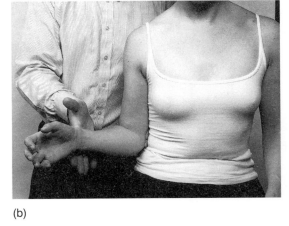

(b)

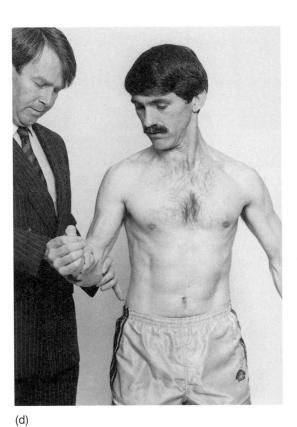

(d)

(c)

Figure 7.16 Resisted (isometric) contraction of (*a*) supraspinatus, (*b*) infraspinatus, (*c*) subscapularis and (*d*) biceps brachii are demonstrated. The examiner notes the presence of pain and/or weakness

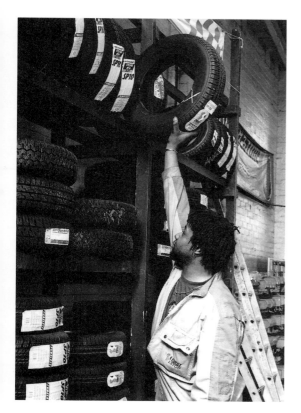

Figure 7.17 Workers engaged in propulsive overhead work may develop chronic multidirectional subluxation

humerus relieves the discomfort and apprehension of anterior subluxation and allows a slightly greater range of passive movement (Figure 7.18c). For the demonstration of posterior instability, the patient should also be examined supine (Figure 7.18d): the humeral head may be subluxed posteriorly when the examiner gently pushes the flexed humerus backwards, and relocated with a clunk or a click on abduction of the arm.

A clicking may be experienced by both the patient and the examiner when the humeral head subluxes or relocates on one of the laxity tests in either anterior or posterior instability.

Palpation
A defect in a torn supraspinatus tendon may be palpated close to its attachment to the greater tuberosity. Similarly, a defect at the musculotendinous junction of the infraspinatus may be palpated posteriorly: this indicates a specific tear of the infraspinatus, and is

probably underdiagnosed (occurring as a result of sport in young adults and as a result of trauma or overload in the middle-aged and elderly).

Tenderness of the respective elements of the rotator cuff may accompany tendinitis. Acute subacromial bursitis (which is commonly a rheumatological condition) is exquisitely tender. Tenderness of the subacromial region is otherwise a common but non-specific feature.

The elbow

Observation
In the severe form of type 2 WRULD the elbow may be held in semi-flexion (see Figure 6.1). Swelling over the olecranon process suggests olecranon bursitis (which is referred to as 'beat elbow', prescribed disease PD A7 in the UK when it is caused by trauma, often repetitive friction, at work). Soft tissue swelling overlying the common extensor origin at the lateral epicondyle may be seen with a moderately severe lateral epicondylitis.

Active and passive movements
Flexion at the elbow is normally 140–150 degrees. Extension is normally 0–10 degrees. (More than this degree of extension is referred to as hyperextension.) There is a soft (tissue approximation) end-feel to flexion, whereas the end-feel to extension should be hard (bone on bone). A springy block to extension may indicate one of a number of pathologies, including an intra-articular loose body, but in the context of WRULDs there may be a 5–10 degrees (springy) loss of extension in the acute form of lateral epicondylitis. Loss of flexion greater than loss of extension is the capsular pattern – usually indicative of osteoarthritis in the chronic case, and synovitis or haemarthrosis in the acute case following trauma.

In the acute stage of lateral epicondylitis, passive palmarflexion of the wrist with the elbow fully extended and the forearm pronated (sometimes referred to as Mills' test (Figure 7.19)) is painful. However, discomfort felt in the proximal forearm on stretching the common extensors in this fashion should be distinguished from discomfort felt over the

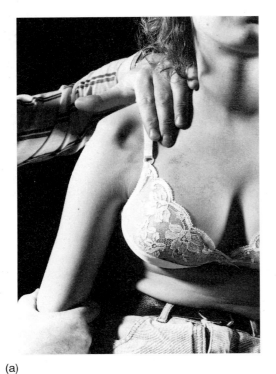

(a)

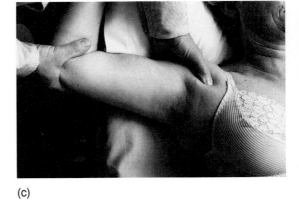

(c)

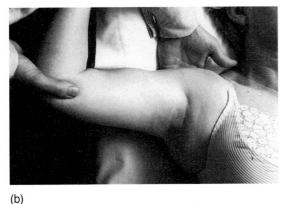

(b)

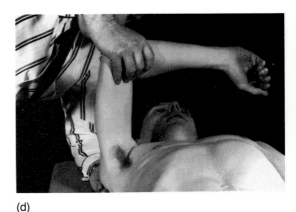

(d)

Figure 7.18 Glenohumeral instability may be demonstrated by: (*a*) inferior laxity; (*b*) anterior apprehension test; (*c*) the Jobe relocation test – the examiner exerts backwards pressure with his thumb on the humeral neck to relocate the head of the humerus; (*d*) posterior stress test. (From Hutson, 1996, by permission).

dorsum of the wrist as the latter indicates wrist pathology such as inflammation of the dorsal wrist tendons, a sprain of the dorsal wrist ligaments, or an occult dorsal wrist ganglion.

The common flexors are stretched by extension of the elbow, supination of the forearm and passive dorsiflexion of the wrist: discomfort is felt along the ulnar and volar aspects of the forearm in medial epicondylitis.

Resisted (isometric) movements

The resisted movements are elbow flexion and extension, and wrist palmarflexion and dorsiflexion (to test those muscles arising from the distal humerus which act over both elbow and wrist). In practice, these are combined with resisted radial and ulnar deviation of the wrist, resisted flexion and extension of the fingers, and resisted pronation and supination of the forearm (see next section). The common extensors are tested specifically by resisted dorsiflexion of the wrist (Figure 7.20), extension of the fingers (Figure 7.21) and radial deviation of the wrist.

Assessment of the musculotendinous structures arising from the medial epicondyle (the 'common flexors') is performed along similar lines. Although it is often stated that resisted wrist flexion is often painful in medial epicondylitis, this is much less common than the observation of pain on resisted pronation of the forearm. Indeed, the latter is virtually pathognomonic of medial epicondylitis.

Palpation

The medial epicondyle, lateral epicondyle and olecranon process are palpated. If tenderness is present, it is usually at the attachment of the common flexors, common extensors and triceps respectively. Occasionally, triceps tendinitis or biceps tendinitis are found at the

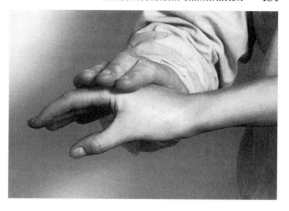

Figure 7.20 Resisted dorsiflexion of the wrist is painful in tennis elbow

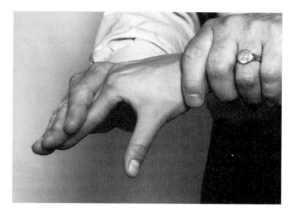

Figure 7.21 Resisted (isometric) contraction of the finger extensors is demonstrated

elbow, and are associated with localized tenderness of the respective tendon close to its insertion and discomfort on resisted contraction, but these conditions are relatively easy to distinguish from the more common tennis elbow (lateral epicondylitis) and golfer's elbow (medial epicondylitis).

On palpating the common extensor origin at the lateral epicondyle of the humerus, it should be recalled that the extensor carpi radialis longus (ECRL) arises from the supracondylar ridge. However, the extensor carpi radialis brevis (ECRP) is the muscle most often affected in lateral epicondylitis, giving rise to the typical exquisite tenderness just anterior to the lateral epicondyle. In medial epicondylitis tenderness is felt approximately

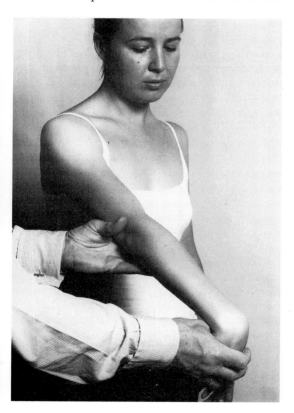

Figure 7.19 Mills' test is demonstrated: pain is reproduced in tennis elbow when the elbow is fully extended, the forearm pronated, and the wrist passively palmarflexed

1 cm distal to the tip of the medial epicondyle on its volar aspect.

Posterior to the medial epicondyle, the ulnar nerve may be palpated in the proximal part of the cubital tunnel. Tinel's sign may be elicited: pressure over the nerve gives rise to paraesthesiae in the ulnar two fingers. The mobility of the ulnar nerve in its tunnel may also be assessed.

Tenderness of the head of the radius may be present in an atypical 'tennis elbow'. On palpating the muscles of the proximal forearm for abnormal tenderness (hyperalgesia), care should be exercised by comparing the painful with the non-painful side. Deep palpation of the common extensor muscles at their anterior margin, some 6–8 cm from the lateral epicondyle, is usually painful in the normal subject. Hyperalgesia affecting both the common extensors and common flexors, 3–8 cm from their elbow origins, is a feature of type 2 WRULD; bilaterality is present in some patients.

The forearm

The movements taking place at the superior and inferior radio-ulnar joints – supination and pronation – are considered in this section. In terms of function, of course, the study of joints in isolation is artificial: manual tasks, at home or at work, require synchronized movements at most, if not all, of the joints of the upper limb. However, the importance of pronation and supination cannot be overstated: loss of rotation severely affects the function of the hand in its various activities such as using a screwdriver, opening bottles and turning door knobs. The positioning of the hand too is dependent upon full rotation of the forearm; the use of a keyboard demands full pronation, although, if restricted, this may be assisted by internal rotation of the shoulder.

Active and passive movements
From the neutral position (with thumb upmost), the patient is asked actively to supinate and pronate their forearm (Figure 7.22). These movements are normally considered to be through 90 degrees (though some 10–15

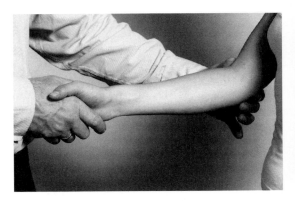

Figure 7.22 From the mid-point of forearm rotation, isometric contraction and the passive range of supination and pronation may be assessed

degrees of this occurs at the wrist). The end-feel is soft. Loss of supination is a frequent consequence of a Colles' fracture at the wrist: this may seriously impair the ability to perform a variety of manual tasks.

Joint play (accessory) movements
I commend the techniques described by John Mennell demonstrating joint play at the inferior radio-ulnar joint (Figure 7.23) (Mennell and Zohn, 1976). Effectively, the distal ulna is moved on the radial styloid; loss of mobility results from injuries affecting the inferior radio-ulnar joint, including Colles' fracture.

Resisted (isometric) movements
Supination should be considerably stronger than pronation; activities such as tightening a screw often require substantial power of supination. Supination is produced by biceps brachii (innervated by the musculocutaneous nerve, C5 and C6) and the supinator muscle (innervated by the posterior interosseous nerve, C5 and C6 too). Very occasionally, supination is weak following an injury, usually traumatic, to the anterior aspect of the elbow, resulting in a neuropraxia of the posterior interosseous nerve. Loss of power of supination also results from rupture of the distal biceps tendon – a particularly serious injury (with respect to function) in a manual worker (Figure 7.24).

Combined discomfort and slight weakness of resisted supination may occur in the radial tunnel syndrome. There is no pain or loss of power of supination in lateral epicondylitis.

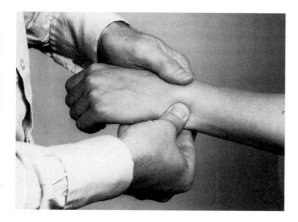

Figure 7.23 To demonstrate joint play at the inferior radio-ulnar joint the distal ulna (grasped by the examiner's right hand in this demonstration) is moved on the radial styloid (which is stabilized by the examiner's left hand)

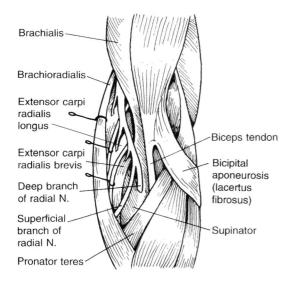

Figure 7.24 Rupture of the distal biceps tendon is a serious injury in a manual worker. The distal attachments of the biceps brachii and the topographical relationships of the radial nerve and supinator muscle are illustrated

Painful resisted pronation (and weakness due to pain inhibition) occurs in medial epicondylitis. In the pronator syndrome, resisted pronation may reproduce the sensory symptoms of median nerve compression. Painless weakness of pronation occurs in the anterior interosseous nerve syndrome.

Palpation

The soft tissues of the forearm are palpated for tenderness. As previously described, muscle tenderness in the proximal forearm is common in type 2 WRULD.

In the distal forearm, palpatory techniques are an important aspect of the diagnosis of intersection syndrome. Tenderness may be detected by gently palpating the intersection between the tendons of extensor pollicis brevis and abductor pollicis longus, and the underlying extensor carpi radialis longus and brevis in the distal forearm. Crepitus is felt when the patient passively palmarflexes and dorsiflexes the wrist: this is commonly associated with localized tenderness and swelling.

The wrist

The ability to stabilize the wrist, a function of the flexors and extensors, and also of abductor pollicis longus, is a prerequisite for normal hand function. Should this ability be lost, for example as a result of a painful tenovaginitis of one of the tendons acting over the wrist, the loss of function of the hand is often severe. These muscles provide active movements at the wrist when the hand is fixed in a grip, for instance when using a light hammer.

Most dynamic activity at the wrist occurs in the transverse plane: ulnar deviation is a vital component of the power grip, and radial deviation may be considered to be a recovery phase of many activities (Figure 7.25). However, when radial deviation requiring the action of abductor pollicis longus is dominant, there is a risk of the development of de Quervain's tenovaginitis. A modest loss of movement at the wrist often gives rise to minimal disability as the full ranges of palmarflexion and dorsiflexion are rarely used for most manual activities.

Observation

Bony deformities of the wrist, particularly those resulting from incomplete reduction of a Colles' fracture, are noted. Soft tissue swellings are more often present over the dorsum of the wrist than over the volar aspect: of

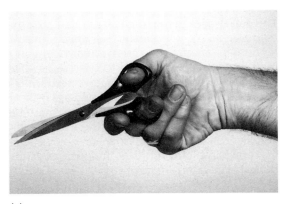

(a)

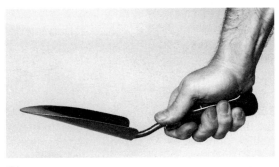

(b)

Figure 7.25 (*a*) Ulnar deviation is the most common functional position of the wrist but (*b*) radial deviation is dominant in some activities

particular relevance are the presence of ganglions and synovial proliferation. When synovial proliferation is diffuse or extensive, and affects the dorsum of the hand, rheumatoid arthritis is the likely diagnosis (see Figure 5.12).

Active and passive movements

The active movements of dorsiflexion, palmarflexion, radial deviation and ulnar deviation are tested in each wrist in turn. These are followed by passive movements in the same directions. Radial and ulnar deviations are assessed with the wrist held straight (in zero flexion); mobility in the transverse plane is much reduced in wrist dorsiflexion and particularly in palmarflexion.

Normal ranges of movement are: palmarflexion 80–90 degrees, dorsiflexion (extension) 70–90 degrees, radial deviation 15 degrees, and ulnar deviation 30–45 degrees. The end-feel of flexion and extension is soft; the end-feel of both deviations should be hard. Loss of both flexion and extension in equal proportions is the capsular pattern at the wrist joint, and usually indicates some type of arthritis. Painful restriction of passive palmarflexion of the wrist as an isolated finding indicates a probable lesion of the tendons acting over the dorsum of the wrist, a ganglion (overt or occult) or a sprain of the dorsal wrist ligaments.

Maintenance of full palmarflexion of the wrist for one minute constitutes Phalen's test for carpal tunnel syndrome. This is commonly performed by asking the patient to fully palmarflex both wrists simultaneously by pressing the dorsum of the hands together (Figure 7.26a). This position should be maintained for fully one minute. The test is positive when tingling and/or numbness are felt in the thumb and adjacent fingers (the sensory distribution of the median nerve).

The reversed Phalen's test – the combination of wrist dorsiflexion, extension of the fingers and forearm supination, is an important test too (Figure 7.26b). This is commonly an uncomfortable position when carpal tunnel syndrome results from underlying tendinitis of the finger flexors. It is a useful pointer to aetiology when the symptoms of carpal tunnel syndrome fail to resolve completely following surgery.

Discomfort on passive radial deviation of the wrist, thereby stretching the tendons that ulnar deviate the wrist, is an important sign in flexor carpi ulnaris tendinitis. The extensor carpi ulnaris tendon may be visualized and palpated close to its insertion on the base of the fifth metacarpal when the dorsiflexed wrist is actively ulnar deviated (Figure 7.27a). In extensor carpi ulnaris tendinitis (Figure 7.27b) discomfort is reproduced on the combination of radial deviation of the wrist and pronation at the wrist/forearm; in my experience discomfort is more marked when this combined movement is performed actively (Figure 7.27c).

Finkelstein described a test in which the wrist is passively ulnar deviated and the thumb is passively opposed across the palm, thereby stretching the EPB and APL tendons (Figure 7.28). Discomfort (a positive test) is experienced by the patient with de Quervain's

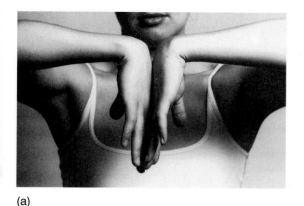

(a)

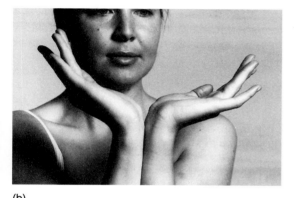

(b)

Figure 7.26 (*a*) Phalen's test is commonly performed by asking the patient to fully palmarflex the wrists by pressing the dorsum of the hands together; (*b*) the reversed Phalen's test requires maintenance of wrist dorsiflexion with finger extension

syndrome. The degree of discomfort is compared with the normal side.

Joint play (accessory) movements

I commend the anteroposterior (AP) glide test described by Mennell and Zohn (1976). The arm should be in a relaxed position, with 45–90 degree flexion of the elbow. AP glide of the proximal row of carpal bones on the distal radius and ulna may be achieved when the examiner stabilizes the distal radius and ulna with one hand and grasps the proximal carpus with the other – the hands should be close together (Figure 7.29). If the examiner moves both hands distally, stabilizing the proximal row of carpal bones with one hand and grasping the distal row with the other, AP glide

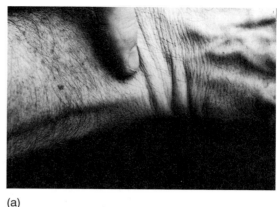

(a)

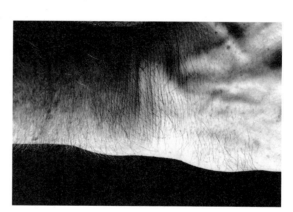

(b)

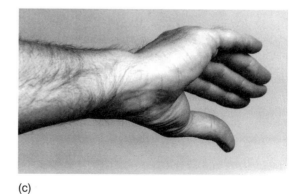

(c)

Figure 7.27 (*a*) Extensor carpi ulnaris is visualized when the hand is dorsiflexed and ulnar deviated at the wrist. (*b*) The swelling of extensor carpi ulnaris tendinitis is seen in profile. (*c*) The combination of radial deviation of the wrist and pronation of the wrist/forearm provokes discomfort in extensor carpi ulnaris tendinitis

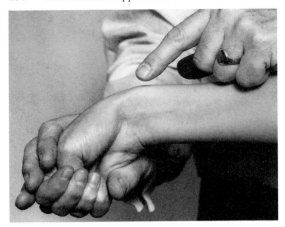

Figure 7.28 Passive ulnar deviation of the wrist and opposition of the thumb constitutes Finkelstein's test. The tendons of the first dorsal compartment of the wrist are clearly seen

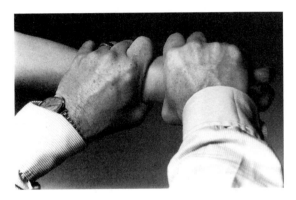

Figure 7.29 The examining position for the assessment of joint play at the carpus is demonstrated

between the two rows may be achieved. Loss of mobility indicates joint dysfunction (commonly found after immobilization of the wrist).

Resisted (isometric) movements
All the muscles acting over the wrist, including those to the thumb, should be tested by isometric contraction (as well as by stretching which has already been described). Tendinitis affecting each group of tendons acting over the wrist has been recorded, although the aetiology may be different in each case. Therefore, it is important for the examiner to resist dorsiflexion, palmarflexion, radial deviation and

ulnar deviation of the wrist as well as the movements of the fingers and thumb. As usual, a note is made of power and discomfort. Weakness may result from loss of innervation (see below, Neurological examination).

Palpation
Palpation of the structures comprising the wrist should be performed gently but methodically. A 'heavy-handed' approach will reveal spurious tenderness (for instance, in the anatomical snuff box).

The dorsal bony landmarks are the radial styloid, Lister's tubercle (of the radius, around which extensor pollicis longus angulates) and the ulnar styloid. Distally, the carpal bones and the dorsal wrist ligaments are palpated, though, in the context of work-related upper limb disorders, there is relatively less information to be gleaned from this examination than in traumatology. The carpometacarpal (trapeziometacarpal) joint of the thumb should be palpated; it may be tender as a result of degenerative changes and enter into the differential diagnosis of conditions such as de Quervain's tenovaginitis that give rise to pain at the base of the thumb and radial aspect of the wrist. Bossing of the base of the second or third metacarpal may be mistaken for a ganglion.

On the volar side of the wrist a number of the carpal bones may be palpated. The pisiform may be moved transversely on the triquetral when the wrist is relaxed in the flexed position (Figure 7.30): pisiform–triquetral compression discomfort is present in 'chondromalacia' or 'sesamoiditis'. Tenderness adjacent to the pisiform is a feature of flexor carpi ulnaris tendinitis. Distal to the pisiform bone is the hook of hamate (the distal ulnar margin of the transverse carpal ligament) which is available to the examining finger on deep palpation. The bony prominence to the volar aspect of the first carpometacarpal joint is the tubercle of the scaphoid (the proximal radial margin of the transverse carpal ligament).

The examiner should then palpate the tendons that cross the wrist. From the radial to the ulnar aspect of the dorsum of the wrist, the extensor tendons are contained within six compartments, all of which are palpable and potential sites for tendinitis (see Figure 5.11).

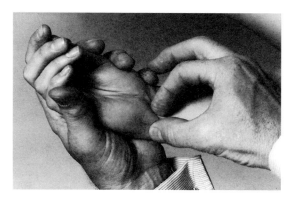

Figure 7.30 The pisiform may be grasped by the examiner and moved transversely on the triquetral when the wrist is relaxed in palmarflexion

1   First dorsal compartment: abductor pollicis longus (APL) and extensor pollicis brevis (EPB).
2   Second dorsal compartment: extensor carpi radialis longus (ECRL) and brevis (ECRB).
3   Third dorsal compartment: extensor pollicis longus (EPL).
4   Fourth dorsal compartment: extensor digitorum and extensor indicis proprius (EIP).
5   Fifth dorsal compartment: extensor digiti minimi (EDM).
6   Sixth dorsal compartment: extensor carpi ulnaris (ECU).

From the radial to the ulnar volar aspect of the wrist, the long flexor tendons are palpated:

1   Flexor carpi radialis
2   Flexor pollicis longus
3   Flexor digitorum sublimis
4   Flexor digitorum profundus
5   Palmaris longus (when present, overlying flexor digitorum sublimis which overlies flexor digitorum profundus)
6   Flexor carpi ulnaris

Careful palpation is necessary to detect localized tenderness and thickening, particularly when tendinitis has passed through the acute stage to become subacute or chronic. Palpation should commence at a point that is not usually tender, gradually moving to areas of particular relevance. As usual, a comparison is made with the normal wrist.

A ganglion may be palpated around the wrist. Although this is most commonly present on the dorsum of the wrist, it may arise on the volar aspect too (see Figure 5.14). On the dorsal surface of the wrist, a ganglion becomes more prominent when the wrist is palmarflexed. The lunate bone becomes more prominent in this position too, and this should be distinguished from a true cystic swelling. Tenosynovitis of the extensor tendons may be associated with a significant degree of synovial swelling; its extent should be recorded.

The hand

Although the hand is used for a wide range of activities, its basic function is to grasp. For this activity sophisticated sensory perception and fine motor control are required. The clumsiness described by sufferers of carpal tunnel syndrome is probably a reflection of the loss of cutaneous sensation in the radial finger pads rather than motor weakness. Motor weakness on the other hand may seriously compromise the various grips, which will be described briefly.

The *power grip* is required for handling many tools (Figure 7.31*a*). All the joints of the hand are flexed but, additionally, there is ulnar deviation and rotation of the fingers to produce obliquity of the grip. There is some degree of flexion and opposition of the thumb at the carpometacarpal (CMC) joint. The power of the grip is dependent upon the long flexors, but injuries to the ulnar nerve, causing loss of intrinsic muscle action, also adversely affect normal grip function.

The *precision grip* is used for more delicate handling of objects, requiring greater tactile appreciation, such as holding a pen or an earring (Figure 7.31*b*). Flexion occurs principally at the second to fifth metacarpophalangeal (MCP) joints, and thumb opposition at the carpometacarpal joint plays an important role. Normal function of both the median nerve and the ulnar nerve is required to activate the small thenar and digital muscles.

The *pinch grip* requires adduction of the thumb and contraction of the first dorsal interosseous muscle (Figure 7.31*c*). A key grip is a type of *lateral pinch grip*, in effect a powered precision grip. Other grips such as the *hook*

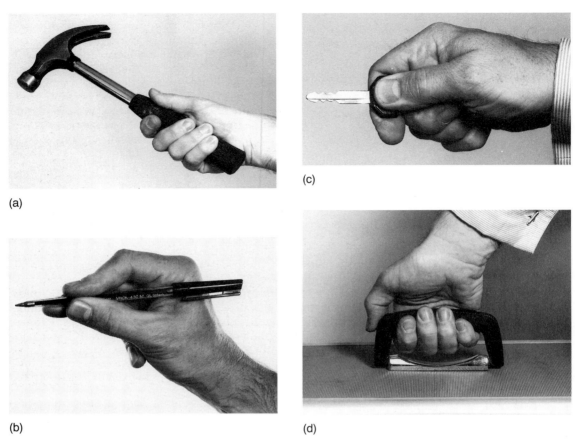

(a)

(b)

(c)

(d)

Figure 7.31 The principal grips are illustrated: (*a*) power grip; (*b*) precision grip; (*c*) lateral pinch (key) grip; (*d*) hook grip

grip, used for carrying a bag or briefcase (Figure 7.31*d*), and the *ball grip* (more commonly used in sport), have less relevance to occupational disorders.

Observation

Neurological deformities such as claw hand, benediction hand or drop wrist are not features of the WRULDs, but wasting of the thenar eminence (in median nerve compression) or hypothenar eminence (in ulnar nerve compression) may be observed if the underlying nerve entrapment has been neglected or misdiagnosed.

The typical 'knobbly' features of nodal osteoarthritis (Figure 7.32*a*) affecting the distal interphalangeal (DIP) joints (Heberden's nodes) are noted. The corresponding deformities at the proximal interphalangeal (PIP) joints are referred to as Bouchard's nodes. The spindle-shaped swellings of rheumatoid arthritis typically affect the proximal interphalangeal joints (Figure 7.32*b*).

Of relevance to the differential diagnosis of pain in the region of the base of the thumb (including de Quervain's tenovaginitis) is osteoarthrosis of the first carpometacarpal (CMC) joint. A lip or ledge may be observed between the first metacarpal and the trapezium, giving a typical 'square hand' (Figure 7.32*c*). Muscle wasting of the thenar eminence may be profound.

The thickening of the palmar fascia associated with Dupuytren's contracture is visible as well as palpable. The fixed flexion contracture at the fourth and fifth MCP and PIP joints gradually becomes profound (see Figure

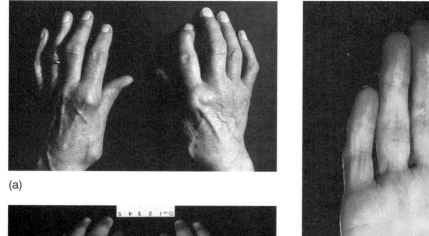

(a)

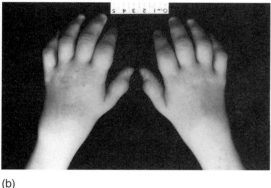

(b)

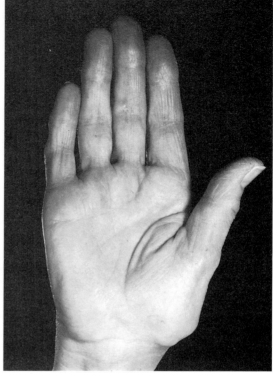

(c)

Figure 7.32 Inspection of the hand may reveal: (*a*) nodal osteoarthritis; (*b*) rheumatoid arthritis affecting the proximal interphalangeal joints; (*c*) osteoarthritis of the first carpometacarpal joint

5.15). Fixed flexion of the fingers may also be observed in chronic flexor tenosynovitis affecting the digits.

Vasomotor changes, such as blueness or swelling of the digits, dystrophic nail changes and increased sweating, may be observed. Occasionally the end changes of reflex sympathetic dystrophy – the shiny atrophic skin of a withered hand – are seen.

Active and passive movements
The patient is asked to straighten the fingers and then to make a fist to demonstrate the movements at the CMC, MCP and IP joints of the thumb and fingers. The capsular pattern of loss of movement at the IP joints, that is seen for instance in the arthritides, is greater loss of flexion than extension.

At the CMC joint of the thumb, at which there is a wide range of movements to allow for manual dexterity as well as power and pinch grips, the capsular pattern in osteoarthritis is more loss of abduction than extension (both of which are painful in the symptomatic subject). These movements are particularly painful when gentle overpressure is applied by the examiner. If there is doubt regarding the diagnosis of osteoarthritis at the CMC joint of the thumb, the provocative tests of 'grinding' or 'cranking' combined with axial loading of the thumb may be performed (see Chapter 5, de Quervain's disease – differential diagnosis).

Ulnar laxity at the first MCP joint (as a result of 'skiers' thumb', for instance, or as a consequence of repetitive stress on the ulnar collateral ligament as in 'gamekeeper's thumb') may be responsible for loss of power of pinch.

Joint play (accessory) movements
Anteroposterior glide, axial rotation and abduction/adduction may be demonstrated

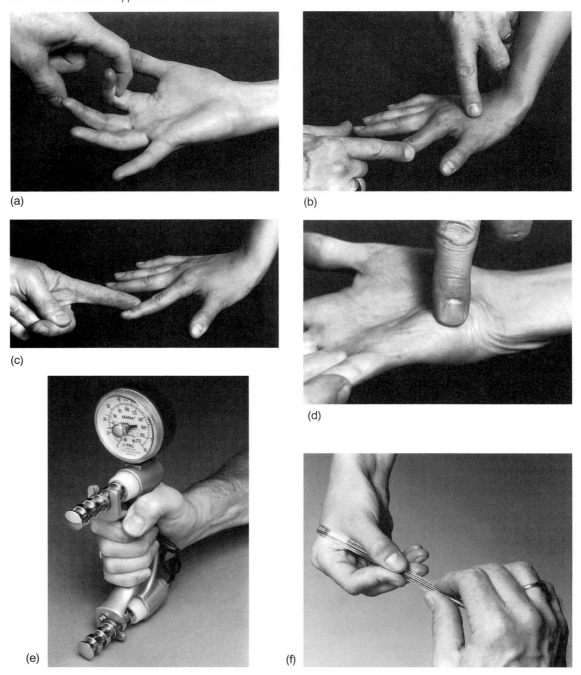

Figure 7.33 Examples of the assessment of muscle power in the hand are shown. (*a*) resisted contraction of the finger flexors; (*b*) resisted contraction of the first dorsal interosseous; (*c*) resisted contraction of the second palmar interosseous; (*d*) resisted contraction of the abductor digiti minimi; (*e*) the use of a Jamar dynamometer for the power grip; (*f*) an attempt to pull a pen away from the patient's grasp for the precision grip; (*g*) an attempt to remove a key or card held by the patient for the pinch grip; (*h*) the use of a pinch gauge for the lateral pinch grip

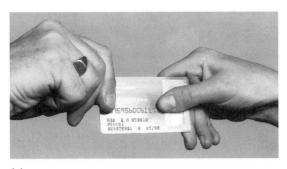

(g)

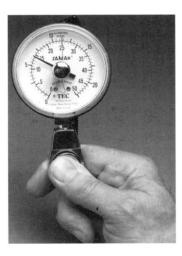

(h)

Figure 7.33 continued

maximally in slight flexion at the MCP joints and full flexion at the IP joints. If the hand needs to be immobilized the MCP joints should be fully flexed and the IP joints of the fingers should be fully extended: there is increased tension in the collateral ligaments and little joint play in these positions, thereby reducing the likelihood of post-immobilization contracture.

Resisted (isometric) movements and grip
Examples of the assessment of muscle power in the hand are demonstrated in Figure 7.33. To assess the physiological function of the long flexors and extensors of the digits, the examiner resists finger flexion and extension. Pain and/or weakness are noted. The power of the intrinsic muscles responsible for finger adduction and abduction is also assessed during a full neurological examination. At the

thumb, the examiner resists flexion, extension, abduction, adduction and opposition.

For a functional assessment of the hand the strength of the power grip, the precision (or prehensile) grip and pinch grip are required. A dynamometer may be used for the power grip (Figure 7.33*e*). The precision grip may be assessed when the examiner attempts to pull a pen or pencil away from the patient's grasp (Figure 7.33*f*). Pinch grip strength may be gauged when the patient grips tightly on a key or card which the examiner attempts to remove (Figure 7.33*g*). A pinch gauge may also be used (Figure 7.33*h*).

Palpation
The thickening of the palmar fascia in Dupuytren's contracture and of the flexor tendon sheath overlying the relevant MCP joint in a trigger digit may be palpated.

Squeeze tenderness at the PIP joint in rheumatoid arthritis may be present. The margins of an arthritic CMC joint of the thumb are often tender. Tenderness of the contractile structures is noted but is uncommon other than for deep tenderness (hyperalgesia) of the muscles in the web between the thumb and forefinger. Triggering may be palpated on release of a trigger finger or thumb.

Neurological examination

Motor function will already have been tested during the previous examination routine. Light touch two-point discrimination establishes the presence of functional sensation required to manipulate small objects (Tubiana, 1984). However, it is contentious as to whether formal sensory examination, for instance by the two-point discrimination test (Figure 7.34) which requires the cooperation of the 'blinded' patient, is of much value. Although an objective assessment of sensory impairment should be included in a comprehensive neurological examination, patients' symptoms are probably a more reliable guide.

Tinel's test applies to any nerve to which pressure is applied by the examiner. In the upper limb, its principal use is at the wrist, where tapping over or pressure upon the median nerve in the carpal tunnel may provoke the sensory symptoms of carpal tunnel

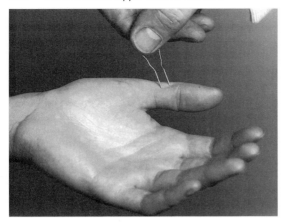

Figure 7.34 The two-point discrimination test is often performed by using a reconstructed paper clip as demonstrated

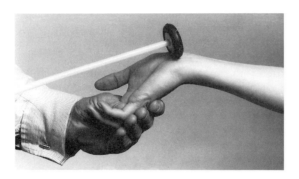

Figure 7.35 The sensitivity of Tinel's test may be increased by using a 'Queen's Square' tendon hammer

syndrome. It is generally considered to be an insensitive test (see Chapter 5), but the sensitivity may be increased by percussing the *extended* wrist over and immediately proximal to the carpal tunnel using a 'Queen's Square' tendon hammer (Mossman and Blau, 1989) (Figure 7.35).

Examination is not complete without assessment of neural tension. Few medical practitioners have been taught or have developed the expertise to apply the brachial plexus tension test (BPTT) or its derivatives – the individual nerve tension tests – but they are useful in the differentiation of somatic and neural disturbances. A particular problem with the conduction of the test(s) is that

patients with type 2 WRULD exhibit allodynia and hyperalgesia on activation of mechano-receptors situated in their connective tissues as well as their nerve roots and peripheral nerves. Accordingly, the interpretation of neural tension tests is difficult unless the examiner is experienced. The tests described by

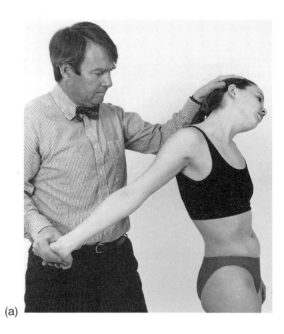

(a)

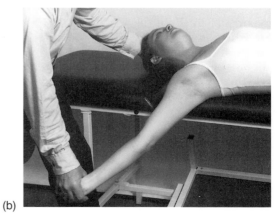

(b)

Figure 7.36 The brachial plexus tension test (BPTT) is demonstrated: depression of the shoulder, extension of the arm at the shoulder, extension of the elbow, supination of the forearm, dorsiflexion of the wrist and contralateral flexion of the cervical spine: (*a*) standing; (*b*) supine

Elvey (1986) are used widely by manipulative physiotherapists.

Although the protagonists of these tests have devised individual stretch tests for the main nerve trunks to the upper limb, I commend the 'basic' test of brachial plexus neural tension – the combination of depression of the shoulder, extension of the arm at the shoulder, extension of the elbow, supination of the forearm, dorsiflexion of the wrist and contralateral flexion of the cervical spine (Figure 7.36). These movements are performed sequentially, thereby gradually increasing the amount of neural stretch. As such, contralateral flexion of the neck is the final movement in the described series (although Elvey preferred elbow extension as the terminal adjustment): discomfort in the arm at this stage (and not merely in the neck) is indicative of positive neural tension.

The test(s) should be performed with the patient relaxed in the supine position. A comparison is made with the normal arm.

References

Bogduk, N. and Marsland, A. (1988) On cervical apophyseal joint pain. In: The cervical zygapophyseal joints as a source of neck pain. *Spine*, **13**, 610–17.

Elvey, R.L. (1986) Treatment of arm pain associated with abnormal brachial plexus tension. *Aust. J. Physiother.*, **32**, 225–30.

Hutson, M.A. (1993) *Back Pain: Recognition and Management*. Butterworth–Heinemann, Oxford.

Hutson, M.A. (1996) *Sports Injuries: Recognition and Management*, 2nd edn. Oxford University Press, Oxford.

Mennell, J. McM. and Zohn, D.A. (1976) *Diagnosis and Physical Treatment: Musculoskeletal Pain*. Little, Brown and Company, Boston, Mass.

Mossman, S.S. and Blau, J.N. (1989) Tinel's sign and the carpal tunnel syndrome. *J. Orthop. Med.*, **11**(3), 72.

Travell, J.G. and Simons, D.G. (1983) *Myofascial Pain and Dysfunction*. Williams & Wilkins, Baltimore, Md.

Tubiana, R. (1984) *Examination of the Hand and Upper Limb*. W.B. Saunders, Philadelphia.

8
Medicolegal aspects

Do Medicine and the Law collude to perpetuate illness
behaviour to the ultimate detriment of our patients?
Reilly *et al.* (1991)

Claims for damages

To achieve success in an action for compensation, a plaintiff has to prove on the balance of probabilities (that is, more likely than not) that an injury was caused by or aggravated by the working conditions; that the development of such an injury or illness was foreseeable; and that the employer has failed in his or her duty of care (in other words, has been negligent). It is noteworthy that there is no burden on the plaintiff to demonstrate that the defendant's negligence was the sole cause of their injury, merely that it was a significant contributory factor (Pheasant, 1994).

In personal injury litigation, medical reports are required to establish the nature of the plaintiff's medical condition, its causation and prognosis. Liability in these cases is not usually an issue that concerns a medical expert, but factors such as excessive workload, lack of job rotation, constrained working postures and poor work environment may be as relevant to the question of liability as they are to aetiology.

In the event that the defendant is found negligent, the plaintiff – the victim of a personal injury – will be able to claim 'special damages' (reflecting pecuniary loss, and including 'reasonable' medical expenses) and 'general damages' (compensation for pain, suffering and loss of amenity).

Medicolegal reporting

A report by the medical expert may be commissioned by the solicitors acting for either party – plaintiff or defendant. The report should be written in good English, to be read and understood by lay people. When necessary, medical terms should be explained.

The opinions expressed in personal injury cases use a 'balance of probabilities' as the *minimum* standard of proof. However, a more firm view (for instance, using a qualification such as 'I have little doubt . . . ') is helpful for clarity if appropriate.

Instructing solicitors doubtless wish a report to present their client's case in as favourable a light as possible. Accordingly, the medical expert may be presented with information or 'advice' that is considered 'helpful'. Lord Wilberforce's comments should be observed: 'While some degree of consultation between experts and legal advisers is entirely proper, it is necessary that expert evidence presented to the Court should be, and should be seen to be, the independent product of the expert, uninfluenced as to form or content by the exigences of litigation' (*Whitehouse* v. *Jordan* [1981] 1 All E.R. 267).

Format of a medicolegal report

The **Introduction** ('Formalities') should include particulars of the patient (full name, address, date of birth), the date and place of examination, the commissioning solicitors, and a list of the documents studied in the preparation of the report.

The **History** should be a comprehensive account of the symptoms, the management by the medical attendants, the investigations undertaken, and the effect on the lifestyle of the plaintiff prior to the date of consultation. A note should be made of the circumstances of the accident, or (particularly with respect to most cases of work-related upper limb disorder) the relationship between the development of the symptoms and the nature of the work activities.

It is often necessary for the examiner to clarify with the plaintiff the ergonomic aspects of the specific tasks undertaken. Although it is not the medical expert's role to give an opinion on the non-medical aspects of the case, background information on work conditions in an individual case is often essential for the formulation of an opinion on causation. This information may be provided in the form of a typed statement by the plaintiff; a videotaped recording may also be made available. Even so, the examiner should record the description of the task given by the plaintiff at interview.

The history should include the present condition in terms of the complaints (physical or psychological), the marital, domestic, or social problems arising, the time lost from work, and the loss of amenity, for instance hobbies, recreational and sporting activities.

The history should also include the past medical history, for which corroboration is often required from the general practitioner's notes and/or the relevant hospital records. In particular, a search should be made for pre-existing medical problems of the same type and for associated conditions which might suggest a systemic or constitutional predisposition or diathesis.

An **Opinion** is based upon the medical expert's knowledge of and experience of the relevant medical condition. A specific (as opposed to a 'syndromic') diagnosis should be made whenever possible.

The opinion should be confined to the medical discipline in which the writer is an expert. Comments upon associated disorders such as psychiatric conditions may need to be qualified by an acknowledgement that this is not the primary field of experience of the expert.

The value placed upon the opinion will, of course, be dependent upon the experience and standing of the medical expert in the medical community.

Of particular relevance to work-related upper limb disorders is the question of causation. The expert should record his or her views on the cause or causes of the medical condition; legally this is referred to as causation. The crux of the question of causation is whether a specific medical condition is attributable to or is not attributable to the effects of the trauma or physical stresses at work. The distinction is often made between a condition of 'constitutional' origin being aggravated by work, and a condition caused by work in an individual who is vulnerable for constitutional reasons. This controversy usually applies to type 1 WRULDs, their causal relationship with work being contested routinely by some experts (except for peritendinitis crepitans which is virtually universally accepted as being directly attributable to repetitive activity). The difference between aggravation and vulnerability may be a fine one, particularly as some conditions have a multifactorial aetiology. In law, for causation to be established in favour of the plaintiff, it is necessary to find that working conditions play a significant part in the development of pain and/or loss of function.

Consideration should be given to the likelihood of the condition arising spontaneously (or for 'constitutional' reasons) and, if so, by what time interval or extent the condition has been advanced or accelerated.

In type 2 (more often than type 1) WRULD, the medical expert may be faced with deciding whether the plaintiff suffers from a genuine medical condition or whether an illness is simulated, fabricated, or substantially exaggerated for the purposes of secondary gain. In this context the expert may have to express an opinion on whether apparently 'inappropriate' behaviour of the patient or 'inappropriate' physical signs on examination (Waddell, 1987) are the result of abnormal illness behaviour (which is probably not a conscious attempt by the patient at fabrication) or the result of malingering.

It will be apparent that neuropathia is the preferred hypothesis for type 2 WRULD in this book. Neuropathic arm pain (NAP) should be considered a genuine medical condition, and distinguished from illness simulation or from somatization. In layman's terms, NAP *should be explained as the development of pain amplification (or sensitization of the central nervous system), often in association with psycho-sociocultural factors, following soft tissue or neural injury.*

The **Prognosis** is an essential component of a medicolegal report. In general it is a prediction of future developments, on a balance of probabilities basis. Consideration should be given to such aspects as:

- the likelihood of, and anticipated timing of, spontaneous resolution;
- the need for further treatment;
- the long-term sequelae – medical, social, psychological, incapacity for work.

Attendance in court

Although the majority of personal injury claims are settled before the matter comes to court, a medical expert should expect to be called to give evidence from time to time. Indeed, any expert should expect to attend court to give evidence each time they write a report.

Accordingly, a report should not be prepared unless it is accepted that it may need to be presented and defended under oath. Medical reports are disclosed, and an opinion on the report of the medical expert (or experts) commissioned by the other side will be requested. If there is much common ground, the experts may not have to attend court. In the event that the reports are not agreed, each side will ask their expert to present their report (and be cross-examined) in court.

The expert is entitled to charge for time and expenses incurred in attending the proceedings.

Judgments of interest

1 Judgment of H. H. Judge John Byrt, 16 December 1991 – *Angela Margaret McSherry and Denise Josephine Lodge* v. *British Telecommunications plc*

The plaintiffs were data processing officers (DPOs) who worked repetitively at key-

boards, with keying speeds up to a minimum standard rate of 10 000 key depressions an hour.

In his preliminary remarks, Judge Byrt accepted that

RSI or work-related upper limb disorder... are terms used to describe generically a number of conditions affecting both muscles and/or their related tendons in the neck, shoulders, and upper limbs which are brought about through their being overloaded as a result of a repetitive stereotype movement. The symptoms might manifest themselves as a well-defined local syndrome [type 1 WRULD in this text] ... or the symptoms might be less well defined, with diffuse aching, weakness, and muscular tenderness brought about by a static or dynamic muscle overloading [type 2 WRULD].

Mrs McSherry suffered from pains that started in her thumbs, working up her arms to her neck, associated with numbness of the middle and ring fingers. Mrs Lodge experienced pain in one hand, radiating to her neck, associated with cramps in the thumb and in the hand.

In his judgment Judge Byrt stated:

I have found that each plaintiff suffered RSI as a result of her work, the condition being brought about by a repetitive stereotype movement of unsupported arms and hands. Further, I have found that strain has been substantially added to by the strains which arose from the *working systems* in place and *poor posture* due to poor ergonomics of the work-station, unsuitable chairs, and, in the case of Mrs. Lodge, the uncorrected bad habits of the operator (my italics).

With respect to the evidence given by the medical experts, he stated 'both consultants agreed that pressures, subjectively experienced by the individual as a response to her work or home environment, her posture, and the ergonomics of her work-station, all added strain to the muscle overload being caused by the work process so as to make the operator the more vulnerable to RSI.

2 Judgment of H.H. Judge Griffiths, 8 July 1991 – *Ping and others* v. *Esselte Letraset Ltd*

The plaintiffs suffered from a variety of specific disorders: epicondylitis, carpal tunnel syndrome, tenosynovitis and tenovaginitis stenosans.

On reviewing these medical conditions, Judge Griffiths stated that:

the evidence shows that those particular pathologies can arise from occupational, constitutional or idiopathic causes and as to the extent to which occupational activities, particularly those involving repetitive movements of the hands and upper limbs, can bring about these conditions [it] is still the subject of much medical controversy, particularly so because such complaints or conditions are common in the general population whether employed or not and most commonly in middle-aged women.

Both Judge Griffiths and Judge Byrt (see previous case) refer to the Health and Safety Executive Guidance Note MS10 (Medical Series 10, 1977) labelling tenosynovitis as the second commonest prescribed disease in the UK. Regulation 34 of the Social Security (Industrial Injuries) (Prescribed Diseases) Regulations 1975 refers to tenosynovitis (subsequently labelled PD A8) as a prescribed, not a notifiable, industrial disease. It is described in the current DSS list of prescribed occupational diseases as 'traumatic inflammation of the tendons of the hand or forearm, or of the associated tendon sheaths'. It occurs in 'any occupation involving: manual labour, or frequent or repeated movements of the hand or wrist'. In addition to tenosynovitis (PD A8), the other prescribed conditions affecting the hand or arm are: cramp of the hand or forearm due to repetitive movements (PD A4), subcutaneous cellulitis of the hand (beat hand) (PD A5), bursitis or subcutaneous cellulitis arising at or about the elbow due to severe or prolonged external friction or pressure at or about the elbow (beat elbow) (PD A7), and carpal tunnel syndrome (as a result of the use of hand-held vibrating tools) (PD A12).

Judge Griffiths judged in favour of the plaintiffs, as 'no warnings were given to the employees and in consequence the defendants were in breach of their duty to give the appropriate warnings and to enforce a proper sense of awareness of the dangers of contracting various work-related upper limb disorders that the plaintiffs in these cases have, in fact, contracted'.

3 Judgment of H.H. Judge Mellor, 9 July 1993 – *Mountenay and others* [9 in all] v. *Bernard Matthews*

Judgment was found in favour of some of the plaintiffs on the grounds of:

(a) the failure of duty of the employer '*to warn*' of the dangers, giving workers an opportunity to make an informed choice as to whether to undertake work which carried a risk of RSI;

(b) failure to implement appropriate *job rotation*;

(c) failure to implement a '*gentle introduction*' to repetitive work.

Of one litigant he stated 'there is ample evidence from witnesses that those who have a previous history of tenosynovitis are disadvantaged in the labour market ... if a worker suffers from a latent disability which would place that worker at a disadvantage in the labour market and a defendant is negligent the plaintiff is entitled to compensation'. Of another litigant he stated that 'workers can suffer RSI without any breach of duty', finding breach of duty was not necessarily causative to what the worker suffered.

Judge Mellor was satisfied that a number of plaintiffs who did not suffer from a recognized condition did, nevertheless, suffer 'beyond normal aches and pains'. Of these plaintiffs he considered that one of the following options may apply:

(a) that they have suffered no pain based on physical conditions but have felt pain as a result of a fixed belief that their conditions have caused the pain;

(b) that there are those whose susceptibility to pain is greater than most might be expected to experience;

(c) that there is some diverse non-specific RSI which may lead to continued disability.

He found in favour of one plaintiff who had carried out repetitive work and had experienced upper limb pain but without evidence of a specific condition. Nominal general damages of £400 were awarded for this case of type 2 WRULD.

4   Judgment of H.H. Judge Prosser, 28 October 1993 – *Mughal* v. *Reuters Ltd*

This hearing, reported as a 'test case', was reputedly the first claim by a keyboard user to be held in the High Court; it was apparently the first by a journalist to reach court; and it was probably the first occasion on which the High Court considered the existence of a type 2 work-related upper limb disorder (Pearce, 1995).

The plaintiff, who worked as a sub-editor for Reuters, claimed that he suffered upper limb symptoms and permanent disability as a result of his work, and that his employers failed to provide him with adequate advice and equipment with which to carry out his job safely.

He was refused damages on the grounds that he failed to convince Judge Prosser that he had suffered 'an injury which he has alleged'. This alleged condition was a repetitive strain injury that was deemed to be a condition unknown to medical science and which did not represent a condition promoted by repetitive work, having neither an identifiable pathology nor an existence as a clinical condition, and accordingly could not form the basis of an action against an employer alleging negligent working methods or environment.

Mistakenly, fuelled by inaccurate press reporting, the impression gained ground that Judge Prosser had denied the existence of any form of RSI or work-related disorder. The failure of the press, and indeed of much of the medical profession, to distinguish between the discrete conditions of known pathology (type 1 in this text) and the 'diffuse condition with no known pathology' (type 2 in this text) by clumping them all under the umbrella term 'RSI' has been responsible for much confusion. In effect, Judge Prosser was saying that he was not persuaded by the medical evidence in this case that type 2 WRULD was a valid diagnosis. No doubt, the views of the judiciary may well change as the understanding of neuropathic pain becomes disseminated more widely.

Conclusions

In the past few years claims for damages for work-related upper limb disorders, both for keyboard operators and for industrial workers, appear to have become more common. Undoubtedly, out of court settlements are the rule in some industries yet are difficult to quantify. According to McDougall, writing in the legal journal *Quantum* (1995), 'patterns of injury are becoming recognized making it easier for the plaintiff to establish foreseeable injury and to claim that unacceptable workplace practices should have been eliminated'. Nevertheless, for a claim for damages to be successful *at the time of writing*, it is necessary to identify a *specific* condition which can be linked to the plaintiff's work.

Reflections

A minority body of medical opinion promotes the concept that the two potentially chronic musculoskeletal conditions of *whiplash injury* to the cervical spine and *refractory occupational arm pain* have a common denominator: illness simulation. The accident neurosis concept of Henry Miller (1961) was applied to 'RSI' in the form of compensation neurosis by Yolande Lucire (1986) and amplified as a conversion phenomenon of 'ills to illnesses', precipitated iatrogenetically by an incompetent medical profession, by David Bell (1989). As a response to the Australian epidemic of 'RSI' there were other opinions too that deprecated the role played by physicians in the perpetuation of the epidemic.

Some authors stop short of defining the condition as illness simulation, preferring to label it as a 'sociopolitical phenomenon', suggesting that the 'majority of sufferers do experience the musculoskeletal symptoms of which they complain and are innocent victims of circumstance rather than seekers of secondary gain' (Ireland, 1988). Others have taken a somewhat more reflective view regarding the role of litigation in the (ill) health of workers. Reilly *et al.* (1991) have posed the questions: 'Do Medicine and the Law collude to perpetuate illness behaviour to the ultimate detriment of our patients? Is disability partly iatrogenic in origin?' Hadler (1985) states that 'once embroiled [in the legal process] it may be difficult to return to health, if such were possible'.

Such cynicism, however just, might be considered to be of secondary sociological importance when compared to the inestimable value of the litigation process in establishing a safe workplace. In some industries effective redress of the discordance between workers' requirements, ergonomic and contractual, and management's obligations demands the continual threat of compensation.

References

Bell, D.S. (1989) 'Repetition strain injury': an iatrogenic epidemic of simulated injury. *Med. J. Aust.*, **151**, 280–84.

Hadler, N.M. (1985) Illness in the workplace: the challenge of musculoskeletal symptoms. *J. Hand Surg.*, **10A**(4), 451–6.

Ireland, D.C.R. (1988) Psychological and physical aspects of occupational arm pain. *J. Hand Surg.*, **13B**(1), 5–10.

Lucire, Y. (1986) Neurosis in the workplace. *Med. J. Aust.*, **145**, 232–6.

McDougall, A.H. (1995) RSI – proving a strain for the plaintiffs? *Quantum*, **2**, 1–3.

Miller, H. (1961) Accident neurosis. *Br. Med. J.*, **i**, 919–25.

Pearce, B. (1995) 'RSI' and the media. *Occup. Health Rev.*, Nov/Dec., pp. 14–18.

Pheasant, S. (1994) Repetitive strain injury – towards a clarification of the points at issue. *J. Personal Injury Litigation*, September, pp. 223–30.

Reilly, P.A., Travers, R. and Littlejohn, G.O. (1991) Epidemiology of soft tissue rheumatism: the influence of the law. *J. Rheumatol.*, **18**(10), 1448–9.

Waddell, G. (1987) A new clinical model for the treatment of low back pain. *Spine*, **12**(7), 632–43.

Index

Page numbers in *italics* represent figures